The Apothecary After the ICU

The

Apothecary After the ICU

One Woman's Journey from the MICU to Natural Healing

and the Tinctures That Changed Everything

— *Briar Hollis* —

First published 2026

ISBN: 979-8-9956856-0-9 (paperback)

Printed in the United States of America

A Note from Dave

In his own words

The last thing I remember before the hospital was telling my wife I couldn't breathe.

I remember trying to get the nurse's attention because I couldn't breathe — yelling and hearing no sound. I thought I was going to die right there. I shook the bed until she came. I remember lying in a hospital bed with people sitting outside my room like they were waiting for me to die.

When I woke up out of the coma, I could not move any part of my body. I tried to talk. Nothing came out. I had no idea where I was. I knew I had gone to the hospital — but I had no idea I was in a different hospital entirely. And I had no idea how long I had been asleep. Not days. Not weeks. Months.

> *They had to suction my lungs out very frequently to remove the blood and clots that were in my lungs. I don't remember thinking about anything in that moment but the sheer terror of no oxygen.*

I remember how hard it was just to sit in a chair. Learning to walk again. Five steps was a good day for a long time.

After weeks of the physical therapy staff and my nurses working with me, getting me stronger and more mobile, one day she came around the corner to visit. I saw her, and something in me clicked.

I just wanted to show her I was going to beat this.

I walked twenty steps that day.

The day I left the medical center, I left by ambulance to the rehabilitation center. I knew I had another month or so ahead of me before I would be able to come home. They played Eye of the Tiger over the loudspeaker through the whole hospital, and there were people lining the halls. I was grateful just to be alive.

Coming home was an amazing moment. And at the same time, I was reduced to someone who could not survive without her one hundred percent support. I could do nothing for myself. That was very hard to accept for a man who was used to being capable.

But with her help, I am able to do many of the things I used to.

If you are reading this book because you are where I was — in that bed, or just home, or somewhere in the long middle of recovery — I want you to know this:

Never give up. You can do anything.

But you need determination. And you need someone even more determined than you are standing behind you.

She was that person for me. Failing was not an option for her. And she made me realize it didn't have to be an option for me either.

Thank you for your support through this tough time, and the continued support to this day. You are truly a faithful and amazing wife.

— Dave

Foreword

This is not a medical textbook. It is not a manifesto against doctors, hospitals, or science. It is something far more personal than any of those things — and far more dangerous to write.

It is the truth.

There is a particular kind of fear that lives exclusively in hospital waiting rooms. It is not the sharp, electric fear of a car accident or a sudden fall. It is slow. It pools. It fills the corners of a room that smells of antiseptic and recycled air, and it waits with you — patiently, unhurried — while machines beep behind closed doors and nurses move past with the practiced calm of people who have seen everything.

I learned to live inside that fear. For a time, I thought I might never leave it.

When the man I love — I will call him Dave, because that is his name, and he has given me permission to tell this story — was admitted to the Medical Intensive Care Unit, I did what most people do in that situation. I trusted the system. I handed him over. I nodded at the things the doctors said and signed the things they put in front of me. And went home each night terrified, falling down rabbit holes looking for answers that the doctors could not give me — too afraid to read all the way to the end.

And then something shifted.

It did not shift dramatically. There was no lightning bolt, no single conversation that changed everything. It was more like a slow turning of light — the kind you notice only in retrospect, when you look back and realize the room you are standing in is nothing like the room you started in. I began asking different questions. Not 'What is wrong with him?' but 'Why is this happening?' Not 'What medication will fix this?' but 'What does the body actually need to heal?'

Those questions led me to plants.

I know how that sounds. I was skeptical too. I had spent decades in a world that equated 'natural' with 'unproven' and 'herbal' with 'wishful thinking.' I had been trained, as most of us have been, to view medicine through a very particular lens — one that privileges the pharmaceutical, the patentable, the clinical trial. And there is real value in that lens. I am not here to throw it away.

But a lens, by definition, shows you only what it is pointed at. And there is an enormous amount of human healing history that modern medicine has simply stopped looking at.

In her landmark work Braiding Sweetgrass, botanist Robin Wall Kimmerer writes about plants as teachers

— beings with their own intelligence, their own relationships, their own gifts to offer if we are willing to pay attention. That framing might feel poetic, even fanciful, to a Western-trained mind. But after two years of living with tincture jars lined up on the counter, of watching Dave's body slowly, stubbornly reclaim its own vitality, I find it less fanciful by the day.

This book is organized in two parts. The first is the story — Dave's story, my story, the story of what happens when a person you love nearly does not make it and you have to decide what kind of healer you are going to become. The second is a reference: an A-to-Z guide to the herbs that became my teachers, organized also by body system and by ailment, so that whether you come to this book in a crisis or out of curiosity, you can find what you need.

I have tried to be honest about what the science says and equally honest about where the science has not yet caught up to centuries of empirical wisdom. I have tried to be fair to the doctors and nurses who kept Dave alive long enough for the herbs to do their work — because that is the truth of it. It was not one or the other. It was both.

Herbalist and author Rosemary Gladstar, often called the godmother of American herbalism, has spent more than five decades teaching people to see the healing potential in the plants growing at their feet. In her foundational book Rosemary Gladstar's Medicinal Herbs: A Beginner's Guide, she writes simply: 'The best herbalist is one who knows the plants.' I would add only this: the best patient is one who knows their options.

I am not a doctor. I am not a licensed herbalist, a naturopath, or a nutritionist. What I am is a woman who watched someone she loves nearly disappear, and then watched him come back — slowly, unexpectedly, with the help of some very old remedies and a great deal of stubbornness on both our parts.

This book is for the people in waiting rooms. For the ones sitting with browsers full of half-read search results and fear that has nowhere to go. For the caregivers and the patients and the skeptics and the quietly desperate.

You deserve more options than you have been offered. These pages are a beginning.

— The Author

Chapter One: Dave

March 23, 2021: The First Hospital

There are things a doctor says to you that you do not fully hear in the moment they are said. You hear the words. You nod. And then you drive home and you do not sleep, and you read about it until two in the morning, and you still cannot make it feel real.

Dave went into the first hospital on March 23, 2021. He had been sick for several days — the kind of sick that starts as something you think you can sleep off and becomes, by degrees, something that changes the quality of the air in the room. He was 60 years old. Strong. Not someone accustomed to being brought low. COVID-19 had other ideas.

The admission was immediate. The isolation was immediate. That was the architecture of COVID hospitalization in the spring of 2021 — you handed your person over at the door, and the door closed, and you went back to your car and sat there for a moment trying to remember how to drive.

I carried most of it alone. Not because people did not love us — family knew, family called — but because there is a particular kind of weight that cannot be distributed. It lives in the body of the person who is there. And I was the one who was there.

The first hospital was ten minutes from home. That proximity was the only mercy of those first days — I could get there quickly, I could leave and come back, the distance was manageable even when nothing else was. The medical center was sixty miles away. When Dave was transferred there on March 31st, everything changed. One hundred and twenty miles, round trip, every single day. The second year of the pandemic had its own rules: one designated visitor only — not one visitor per day, one person for the duration. No rotating family members, no friends taking turns. One person. I was that person, and I was grateful beyond measure to be allowed in at all. The first year of the pandemic, families could not get in at all. I have thought often about those people — who lost someone without being allowed to be present. I cannot fathom how they survived it. I drove down alone. In the beginning, I drove both ways in tears. Sometimes I listened to spiritual music and prayed the entire sixty miles. Sometimes I drove in absolute silence, somewhere beyond what tears or words could reach, the road and the white lines the only things my mind could hold. And sometimes I called his brother, or one of his close friends — the people who loved him the way I did, who needed to hear my voice as much as I needed to hear theirs. Those people hold a permanent, irreplaceable place in my heart. Visiting hours at the first hospital were two to six in the afternoon — the same window I would keep at the medical center for the months that followed. Four hours a day. I gowned up every time — gown, two pairs of gloves, booties, mask, face shield — and I went in and I sat with him. He was intubated. He was in a medically induced coma. I pressed play on our playlist — the songs we had sent back and forth to each other over the years, the ones that meant I am thinking of you without having to say it — and I let them fill the room.

Now they were the only way I had to reach him.

I talked to him. I do not remember exactly what I said. I just remember saying it — keeping my voice steady, then not keeping it steady, then finding it again. And then one day, while I was holding his hand — my gloved hand around his, the latex between us the only barrier I could not dissolve — and the music was playing and I was sobbing, tears ran down his face.

Just like that. From somewhere underneath all of it — the sedation, the machinery, the medically managed silence — his body found a way to respond. He could hear me. Some part of him, in that room full of equipment and protocol and the hum of ventilators, knew I was there.

That broke me. And it also, somehow, held me together.

I felt hopeless in those days in a way I had never felt before — the specific, nauseating helplessness of loving someone who is very sick and having no knowledge of how to fix them. I was not a nurse. I was not a doctor. I could not read the monitors or interpret the labs or ask the right questions in the right language. I could play our music. I could hold his hand through two pairs of gloves. I could come back the next day.

And I could read.

The nights were long and the internet was open and I read everything I could find. About COVID-19 and bilateral pneumonia and what happens to lungs under prolonged mechanical ventilation. About the medications they were giving him and what they did to the liver and the gut and the microbiome. About the body's own capacity to heal, and the conditions under which it does its best work.

One night — the night of March 30th, though I did not know yet why it mattered — I found myself reading about ECMO.

March 31, 2021: The Transfer

The doctor called while I was already in the car, driving to the first hospital for the day's visit.

They needed to transfer Dave to the medical center. He needed ECMO — extracorporeal membrane oxygenation, the machine I had been reading about the night before, the one that removes blood from the body, oxygenates it outside the lungs, and returns it. It is used when the lungs have stopped being able to do that work themselves. It is, in the hierarchy of medical interventions, close to the last option.

I already knew what the word meant. I did not yet know what it would mean for us.

I kept driving to the first hospital. I spoke to the doctor again there, in person. I spent as much time as they allowed with him. I watched his chest rise and fall one more time in that room, with that particular light and that particular sound, before they prepared him for transport.

They called me when he left.

It was at night. I went home. I did not sleep. At some point before the sun came up, the phone rang again — the medical center, telling me what room he was in, what time I could come.

I lay in the dark and listened to them tell me where he was. Outside, the world was still

The Long Middle: The Medical Center

The procedures list on Dave's discharge paperwork from the medical center is three pages long. I have read it many times since, the way you re-read something that does not seem fully real.

It still says the same things every time. ECMO initiated March 31st. Emergency intubation confirmed. A tracheostomy on April 20th — a surgical airway through the front of his throat, because the ventilator tube had been in so long that leaving it was no longer viable. Endobronchial valves inserted into both upper lung lobes to seal the places where air was escaping. Dialysis, because the kidneys had begun to fail. A cardiac event on April 17th that required restoration of rhythm. More than seventeen bronchoscopies over five months. Chest tubes. Blood transfusions. Pleurodesis.

I learned all of these words. I wrote them down. I asked questions and went home and looked things up and came back and asked more questions. I became, over those months, a person with a working vocabulary in a language I had never wanted to learn.

While Dave was on ECMO, he developed sepsis and candida in the bloodstream. He battled both for weeks. The response was systematic — every IV line, every catheter placement was changed to eliminate the source. Everything that could be moved was moved. The one thing they could not change was the ECMO itself. That line stayed. It had to. And so they managed around it, fighting infection in a man whose life depended on a machine they could not touch.

There were four moments — at minimum — when I was told that Dave might not survive. Four separate conversations, with doctors and nurses both, in which someone looked at me and told me, with varying degrees of gentleness, to prepare myself. Four times I nodded and drove home and did not prepare myself at all.

Preparation, I have since decided, is not something you can do in advance for this. What you can do is find something to do with your hands.

> *I started reading about reflexology. About how the soles of the feet are mapped, in traditional practice, to every organ and system in the body. I could not fix his lungs. But I could put my hands on the part of him that connected to them.*

And so I did. Every visit, every day, for as many minutes as I had. I sat at the foot of his bed and worked the points that corresponded to his lungs, his kidneys, his heart. I did not know if it was doing anything. I knew that doing nothing was not an option I was willing to accept.

Reflexology is ancient — documented across cultures from traditional Chinese medicine to Egyptian papyri to the work of American physiotherapist Eunice Ingham, whose 1938 book Stories the Feet Can Tell established the modern Western framework for the practice. A 2011 systematic review in Complementary Therapies in Medicine found modest evidence of benefit for anxiety and quality of life, while calling for more rigorous study.

I am not asking you to believe it fixed him. I am telling you it was the first moment I understood what this book would eventually be about: the refusal to be helpless. The insistence on bringing something — any knowledge, any practice, any tradition that had survived because it helped — into the room.

And somewhere in those long nights at home, between the four hours of sleep and the phone within arm's reach, the reading that had started with ECMO and reflexology began to widen. I found myself in the world of herbs.

Phase Two: Rehab

On August 9, 2021 — four and a half months after his admission to the first hospital — Dave was transferred to a rehabilitation facility. He left the medical center alive. He left with a tracheostomy, with lungs that had survived things lungs were not designed to survive, with a body that had shed an enormous amount of weight and muscle and baseline function.

He left, and I followed.

The second day he was there, he developed a painful rash. Shingles. His immune system, depleted beyond anything it had ever been asked to withstand, had allowed a dormant virus to surface. It was one more thing on top of everything else — treated, managed, added to the list. That is what recovery from something like this actually looks like. It is not a straight line toward better. It is better, and then this, and then better again.

Visiting hours at rehab ran from four to six. I went every day except one — a day I spent at the house preparing it for his return, making it into a place a man on oxygen equipment with limited stamina could actually live in. I FaceTimed him that afternoon instead. I remember apologizing. He told me not to be ridiculous.

It was during these months that my herbal research began to take on specific shape. At the hospital it had been reflexology — touch, presence, the physical language of care when medicine had run its course for the day. At rehab, with Dave now awake and present and visibly struggling, I began thinking about what I could actually give him.

His lungs were the obvious starting point. Chronic respiratory failure was now a formal diagnosis. He had left the MICU on supplemental oxygen. His breathing was labored and effortful — a strong man, working hard for something the rest of us do without thinking.

I started reading about Mullein. The ancient Greeks used it for lung ailments. European herbalists of the medieval period used it. It appears in the traditional medicine of dozens of cultures across as many continents, always for the same purpose — to soothe inflamed airways, to support the lungs in clearing what they cannot clear alone, to make the slow work of breathing a little less hard.

There is something in that continuity that I find deeply reassuring. When you are watching someone fight to breathe after bilateral bacterial pneumonia and five months on a ventilator, the knowledge that human beings have been reaching for a particular plant in exactly that situation for two thousand years is not nothing. It is, in fact, quite a lot.

Phase Three: Home

Dave came home on September 2, 2021. He walked through the door on his walker — steady, deliberate, upright. That walker was not a defeat. It was a man who had been on his back for five months choosing to come home on his own two feet, whatever support that required. He came home with an oxygen concentrator, portable oxygen tanks, and a portable ventilator — not just for sleeping, but with him all the time. The ventilator went where he went. It was the constant companion of those early weeks at home, the hum of it as familiar as any sound in the house. I want to tell you about the day we called to have it picked up. Because there came a day when he did not need it anymore — when the lungs that had failed so completely that he had been on ECMO for months had rebuilt themselves enough that the portable ventilator was no longer necessary. I called the company to arrange the pickup. And the representative on the phone paused and said: we don't get calls like that. That day, they did. I am grateful for that ventilator in the way you are grateful for something that kept someone alive when nothing else would. But I am more grateful for the day we gave it back. He came home careful in his movements, tiring quickly, needing help with things he had done without thought his entire adult life.

He also came home alive.

I want to be careful here, because this is the part of the story where it would be easy to pivot toward a clean redemption narrative — nature healing what medicine could not. That is not what happened. The doctors and nurses at the first hospital and the medical center kept Dave alive through interventions that no herb on earth could have replicated. ECMO is not something you make in a mason jar. A bronchoscopy is not a tincture. I am not here to pretend otherwise.

What I am here to say is that conventional medicine saved his life and then, as it so often does, handed him back to us with a list of follow-up appointments and a prescription bag and very little guidance about what comes next.

> *The discharge paperwork was twelve pages long. Not one of those pages told me how to help him breathe better. Not one mentioned what months of antibiotics, antivirals, and immunosuppressants had done to his gut, his liver, his microbiome. Not one of them asked what he was eating.*

That silence — the silence after the crisis, when the machines are gone and the monitors are gone and it is just the two of you in a house with a concentrator humming in the corner — that is where this book truly begins. That is where the tinctures came in.

Mullein first, for his lungs. Then Burdock Root and Milk Thistle, for the liver bearing the cumulative burden of six months of pharmaceutical intervention. Then Chamomile, for the anxiety and fractured sleep that are nearly universal in MICU survivors — a phenomenon now formally recognized as Post-Intensive Care Syndrome, or PICS, encompassing the physical, cognitive, and psychological aftereffects of critical illness.

Then rose petals, for their gentle support of the heart and immune system — and because sometimes the body needs something as simple and ancient as a flower. Then, gradually, others — each chosen not at random but in response to a specific need, a specific gap between what Dave's body had been through and what his discharge paperwork had offered us.

I was not replacing his pulmonologist. I was not canceling cardiology. I was filling in the space between appointments — the vast, mostly unaddressed territory of what a body actually needs to rebuild itself after something like this.

I had felt hopeless in that room at the first hospital because I had no knowledge of how to fix him. This book is what happened when I decided to get some.

Dave is, at the time of this writing, doing remarkably well. He still carries what he went through — the lungs do not forget five months on a ventilator, and the body does not simply erase six months of critical illness. But he is here. He is breathing. He is himself.

Chapter Two: Coming Home

September 2, 2021

Nobody tells you about the numbness.

They tell you about the joy — the tears, the embraces, the relief of the crisis finally ending. They tell you about the hard work of recovery and the importance of follow-up appointments and the medications to manage and the signs to watch for. What they do not tell you is that a person who has been running on adrenaline for six months, who drove 120 miles every single day to sit beside that bed, who held it together in parking lots and on the side of the road when the doctor called with news she could not fully hear, who drove in tears and in silence and with spiritual music playing and prayed the entire way — that person, when the thing she had been fighting toward finally happens, may feel almost nothing at all.

Not because the love is gone. Not because the relief is not real. But because the body keeps its own accounts, and by September 2, 2021, mine were empty.

Dave came home.

I remember the concentrator being ready. I remember the oxygen tanks positioned where they needed to be. I remember that I had spent the one day I missed visiting him at the rehab facility setting everything up — what he would need downstairs during the day, what he would need upstairs at night, his regular bed modified to accommodate the equipment, the pathways clear, the house reorganized around the shape of his recovery. I had been planning this day for weeks, maybe longer. The house was ready.

I am not sure I was.

> *He had been gone for one hundred and sixty-three days. And when he walked through the door, I felt the full weight of every one of them settle into my body all at once — not as grief, not as joy, but as a kind of vast, quiet exhaustion that had nowhere left to hide.*

I hugged him carefully, the way you hug someone whose body you have learned to be gentle with. I showed him what I had set up. I made sure he was comfortable. And then I went to the kitchen and I stood there for a moment, alone, and I breathed.

That is what I remember most about the day Dave came home. Not the moment itself, but the breath afterward. The first one in six months that did not carry the weight of a hospital room.

The Shape of Recovery

What nobody prepares you for — what the twelve pages of discharge instructions do not cover, what the follow-up appointment scheduler does not mention — is that bringing someone home from a long hospitalization is not the end of the emergency. It is the beginning of a different one. Quieter. Slower. Without monitors or nurses or the reassurance of machines that beep when something goes wrong.

Just you, and him, and the concentrator humming in the corner.

Dave's recovery was not linear. I want to be honest about that, because the literature on Post-Intensive Care Syndrome — PICS, the formal name for the constellation of physical, cognitive, and psychological aftereffects that follow prolonged critical illness — describes exactly this: a recovery that does not move in a straight line, that has good weeks and hard weeks, that can look from the outside like progress and feel from the inside like standing still.

Some days he was frustrated — with his body, with its limitations, with the distance between who he had been and who he was now. Some days he was quieter than his usual self, still processing somewhere deep inside what his body had been through while his mind was under. Some days he surprised me, doing something I had not expected him to be able to do yet, moving through the house with a steadiness that made me catch my breath.

Week by week, he got stronger. Not every week. Not in every direction. But over time, in the way that the tide comes in — so gradually you cannot see it moving, until you look back and realize the shore has changed.

I watched him the way I had watched the monitors at the medical center — constantly, quietly, cataloguing. Looking for the numbers to move in the right direction. Learning to read a different set of signals now that the machines were gone.

The Kitchen Begins to Change

It started with the Mullein.

I made the tea in the kitchen — measured the dried leaves I had harvested from the yard into a cup, poured the boiled water over them, covered it to keep the volatile compounds from escaping with the steam, strained it carefully through a coffee filter to catch every last fine hair. Carried it to wherever Dave was resting. Set it down in front of him.

He looked at it. He looked at me.

He knew, by then, that I had been reading. He knew I had been building something during those months — a protocol, a body of knowledge, a conviction that what his discharge paperwork had given us was not enough. He did not fully understand it yet. He did not ask many questions.

That was enough. That was everything.

He drank the tea.

Over the weeks and months that followed, the kitchen began to transform. Slowly at first — a jar of dried Mullein here, a bottle of Milk Thistle tincture there. Then more deliberately, as I understood better what his body needed and in what order. Burdock Root decoctions simmering on the stove three times a week, filling the house with a deep, earthy smell that Dave eventually came to associate with getting better. Chamomile steeping in the evenings for the anxiety and the fractured sleep. Rose petals in a jar on the windowsill, their faint sweetness a small, deliberate act of beauty in a house that had been very serious for a very long time.

The tinctures came from the farm — small, dark bottles labeled by my farmacy — the farm I had found and come to trust, whose labels I recognized on sight, each one a concentrated extraction of something grown in soil tended by people who knew exactly what they were doing. I lined them up on the counter in the order Dave took them. It started to look less like a

25

kitchen and more like something else. An apothecary, maybe. Or a promise.

I remember standing at the counter one morning, looking at what I had assembled, and thinking: how did I get here? Six months ago I did not know what silymarin was. I did not know what a decoction was. I did not know the difference between a tincture and an infusion or why it mattered. I had learned all of it in the dark, between four-hour stretches of sleep, with the phone within arm's reach and my ears tuned to the frequency of bad news.

And somehow, without planning it, I had built a medicine cabinet.

What PICS Looks Like From the Inside

Post-Intensive Care Syndrome is a relatively recent formal recognition of something caregivers and survivors have known for as long as people have survived ICUs: that leaving the hospital does not mean leaving the illness behind. The physical sequelae — muscle weakness, respiratory compromise, fatigue that does not respond to sleep — are the most visible. But the cognitive and psychological dimensions are equally real and far less discussed.

Dave experienced what many MICU survivors experience: a brain that did not quite work the way it had before. Not dramatically, not in ways that would show on a scan, but in ways he noticed and I noticed. The word that would not come. The train of thought that derailed. The difficulty concentrating on things that had previously required no effort. Researchers call this post-intensive care cognitive impairment, and studies suggest it affects up to 80 percent of MICU survivors to some degree, with effects that can persist for months or years.

The psychological dimension — the anxiety, the hypervigilance, the disrupted sleep — is equally well documented. A significant percentage of MICU survivors meet criteria for PTSD, depression, or anxiety disorders in the year following discharge. The body that went through what Dave's body went through does not simply reset. It carries the memory of what happened to it in ways that take time, and patience, and the right support, to begin to release.

This is where Chamomile came in. And Lemon Balm. And the rose petals on the windowsill. Not as cures for what are genuinely complex neurological and psychological sequelae — Dave also worked with his medical team on this — but as daily, gentle, consistent signals to the nervous system that the emergency was over. That it was safe, now, to begin to soften.

The nervous system, it turns out, does not take anyone's word for this. It has to be shown, repeatedly, over time. Every cup of Chamomile is a small lesson.

Every evening ritual, every moment of deliberate calm, every herb chosen for its capacity to quiet rather than stimulate — these are not luxuries. They are rehabilitation, in the truest sense of the word.

The Protocol Takes Shape

I introduced things slowly. That was deliberate. A body that has been through six months of intensive pharmaceutical intervention is not a body to overwhelm with a dozen new compounds simultaneously. I added one herb at a time, watched for a week or two, noted what seemed to help and what seemed neutral, then added the next.

Mullein first, for the lungs. Always the lungs first — because breathing is everything, because chronic respiratory failure is not a minor diagnosis, because every cell in the body depends on oxygen and Dave's cells had been fighting for it for months.

Then Milk Thistle and Burdock Root together, for the liver. These two I introduced in the second week, as a pair — Milk Thistle protecting and regenerating liver cells, Burdock supporting the lymphatic drainage that helps the liver do its job. They are complementary in the way that good things often are, each one making the other more effective.

Then Chamomile in the evenings, steeped long and drunk slowly, for the nervous system. For the sleep that came in fragments. For the body learning, cautiously, to stand down.

Then rose petals — because the heart had been through something too, in every sense of that word, and because beauty is not frivolous when someone is healing. Because sometimes the medicine is also just something lovely.

Then, gradually, others. Each one introduced with intention. Each one chosen for a specific reason, a specific gap between what Dave's body needed and what his discharge paperwork had offered us.

> *The protocol was not a fixed thing. It was a conversation — between me and the herbs, between the herbs and Dave's body, between what I was learning and what I was observing. It changed as he changed. That is how it is supposed to work.*

A Note for the Caregiver Reading This

If you are reading this chapter because someone you love has just come home from a long hospitalization — or is about to — I want to speak to you directly for a moment, outside of Dave's story.

You are probably exhausted in a way that does not have a name yet. You have been holding things together for so long that holding things together has become your entire identity, and now the crisis is technically over and you do not quite know what to do with your hands.

Here is what I want you to know: the numbness is normal. The flatness is normal. The strange grief of getting what you prayed for and feeling less than you expected to feel — that is normal. It is what happens when a body that has been in survival mode for months is suddenly told it is safe. It does not celebrate. It collapses, very quietly, and begins the long process of remembering how to feel ordinary things.

Give yourself the same patience you are giving the person you brought home. They are not the only one recovering.

And when you are ready — when the concentrator is humming and the tinctures are lined up and you are standing in your kitchen wondering how you got there — know that you got there the same way anyone gets anywhere worth going. One day at a time. One cup of tea at a time. One small, stubborn act of love after another, until love became knowledge, and knowledge became this.

The herb profiles that follow are organized the way my protocol was organized — not alphabetically at first in my mind, but by urgency, by body system, by what Dave needed most and when. The A-Z structure of the reference section is for ease of use. But if you want to understand the order in which I reached for things, Chapter One and this chapter are your guide.

Start with the lungs, if that is where the need is. Start with the liver, if that is where the burden is. Start with the nervous system, if that is where the fear lives. Start somewhere. The body is waiting.

Chapter Three: Home as Medicine

There is a question I kept returning to in the months after Dave came home, as I was reading about herbs and detoxification and liver function and the lymphatic system. It was not a complicated question. It was almost embarrassingly simple.

If we spend all this effort cleaning the organs — if we give the liver Milk Thistle and Burdock Root, if we support the lymph, if we coax the gut back to health with sourdough and bone broth and carefully chosen herbs — and then we fill the body back up with the same things that burdened it in the first place, what exactly have we accomplished?

The answer, I decided, was nothing. Or at least, not nearly enough.

This realization led me somewhere I had not expected to go. I had started with herbs. I thought herbs were the protocol. But the more I understood about how the body processes its environment — not just what we eat, but what we breathe, what we absorb through our skin, what we heat our food in, what we wash our clothes with — the more I understood that the protocol was much larger than a row of tincture bottles on a kitchen counter.

The protocol was the house.

And the house, it turned out, did not belong only to Dave. It belonged to all of us.

My daughters were seven and twelve when Dave went into the hospital in March 2021. They were there when he came home in September — helped me get him inside, helped get him situated, saw with their own eyes the distance between the man who had left and the man who returned. That was a lot for children to hold. They held it anyway, the way children do when the adults around them are holding things too — quietly, without being asked, watching everything.

Those girls are the best. That is not a small thing to say. It is the most precise thing I know.

What happened over the months that followed was not something I planned for them. I was focused on Dave — on the tinctures and the food and the air and the slow, uneven work of rebuilding a body that had been through the unsurvivable. But they lived in the same house. They ate the same food. They breathed the same air. And somewhere along the way, without a family meeting or a lecture or a chart on the refrigerator, the protocol became theirs too.

I want to be honest about how this happened. It was not a single dramatic decision. It was a gradual unfolding over weeks — one realization leading to the next, one cleared shelf leading to another. It started with Dave's food and it ended, several months later, with me standing in the bathroom holding a tube of conventional toothpaste and thinking: this too.

I went, as I have told people since, completely nuts. And I would do it again without hesitation.

The Pantry: Starting from Zero

The pantry went first. All of it, at once. I did not gradually use up what we had and replace it with better options. I cleared it. Boxes, cans, packages — anything with an ingredient list longer than five items or containing a word I could not trace to a farm or a field.

What came out of that pantry was a catalogue of the modern food system at its most convenient and most compromised: seed oils with oxidation rates that make them pro-inflammatory before they even reach the pan; refined sugars that spike insulin and feed the pathogenic organisms we were trying to clear; artificial preservatives that extend shelf life by inhibiting biological processes — the same biological processes the body relies on to heal. Synthetic dyes. Emulsifiers. Flavor enhancers that have no business being in food.

Every one of those pantry items was asking something of Dave's body that his body could not afford to give. And quietly, without making a separate announcement about it, I realized they were asking the same of my daughters. Of me. Of everyone sitting at that table.

So they left.

What replaced them was simple to the point of being almost radical in a modern kitchen: meat from a local farm — chicken and beef raised without hormones or antibiotics, on pasture, by people whose names we know. Organic produce. Farm eggs with yolks so orange they look like small suns. Olive oil. Butter from grass-fed cows. Raw honey. Dried herbs. And the ingredients for bone broth, which became a weekly ritual and one of the most healing things we made.

Bone broth deserves a moment here. It is not a trend. It is one of the oldest foods in human history — the long, slow simmering of bones to extract collagen, gelatin, glycine, proline, and minerals that are bioavailable in a way that no supplement fully replicates. Collagen supports the gut lining, compromised by antibiotic use. Glycine is one of the primary amino acids used in liver detoxification. The minerals — calcium, magnesium, phosphorus — are absorbed more readily from broth than from almost any other source.

We made it every week. We drank it plain. We cooked everything in it. It became, quietly, the foundation of the kitchen.

The kitchen, in turn, became something else entirely. It became the place everyone wanted to be. My daughters — teenagers, which is to say people specifically designed by nature to be anywhere but where their mother is — started hanging around in there. Watching. Asking questions sometimes. Just being present in a room that had become the center of something they could feel even if they couldn't name it yet.

Sourdough: Medicine You Bake Yourself

I started making sourdough bread because of the gut. Not because I had always wanted to bake, not because I had time on my hands — I did not — but because I had read enough about the gut-associated lymphoid tissue to understand that what happens in the gut does not stay in the gut.

The gut-associated lymphoid tissue, or GALT, is the largest component of the entire human immune system. Approximately 70 percent of immune function resides in the gut. The lymphatic vessels that run through the intestinal wall are among the most active in the body, constantly sampling the gut environment and calibrating the immune response accordingly. Feed the gut well, and you are feeding the immune system. Damage the gut — with antibiotics, with processed food, with the stress of prolonged illness — and the consequences ripple outward into every system in the body.

Commercial bread is not bread in any traditional sense. It is flour, water, and a collection of additives assembled in hours rather than days, optimized for shelf life rather than nutrition. The long fermentation that real sourdough requires — 12 to 24 hours or more — is not just flavor development. It is a transformation. Wild yeasts and lactobacillus bacteria break down phytic acid, partially break down gluten proteins, produce lactic and acetic acids that lower the glycemic index significantly, and create a living ecosystem of beneficial organisms that contribute to your own gut microbiome when you eat them.

> *Real sourdough, made slowly and with good ingredients, is a fermented food. It belongs on the same shelf as kefir and sauerkraut — not in the bread aisle next to something that expires in three weeks.*

I learned to make it. I am still making it. The feeding of the starter each morning, the mixing, the long rise, the moment the scored loaf goes into the Dutch oven and the house fills with a smell that is ancient and deeply right — it is one of the most satisfying things I do. My daughters noticed that smell before they noticed anything else changing. Food that smells like it was made by a person, in a kitchen, with real ingredients — the body recognizes it. Even a teenager's body. Especially a teenager's body.

The Air: What We Were Breathing

I removed the candles. All of them.

The majority of scented candles are made from paraffin wax — a byproduct of petroleum refining. When burned, paraffin releases benzene and toluene, both classified as known carcinogens by the EPA. The synthetic fragrance oils in most commercial candles contain phthalates — endocrine-disrupting compounds — along with dozens of other volatile organic compounds that contribute to indoor air pollution.

Air fresheners are worse. They do not clean the air. They introduce a cocktail of synthetic chemicals to mask odor with something that smells pleasant but is itself a pollutant. A study by the Natural Resources Defense Council found phthalates in 12 of 14 common air freshener products, including some labeled as all-natural.

For a man breathing through lungs that had been on a ventilator for five months — burning paraffin and synthetic fragrance in the living room was simply not something I was willing to do. The candles went. The air fresheners went. The house smelled like food, and clean laundry, and herbs steeping on the stove. That turned out to be enough. More than enough. For everyone in it.

The Kitchen: Cookware, Storage, and What Touches the Food

The Teflon pans went next. Polytetrafluoroethylene begins to break down above 500 degrees Fahrenheit, releasing particles and gases associated with flu-like symptoms in humans and lethal to pet birds. The manufacturing of non-stick cookware historically involved perfluorooctanoic acid — PFOA — a compound so persistent it has been detected in cord blood of newborns on every continent. The industry has phased out PFOA, replacing it with compounds whose long-term safety profiles are not yet established. I decided not to wait for that research.

Cast iron and stainless steel replaced the non-stick. Cast iron adds small amounts of dietary iron to food — relevant for anyone recovering from the blood loss and transfusion history that Dave's records showed. The plastic food storage became glass. Glass is inert. It has been holding human food safely for thousands of years without releasing anything into it.

One More Thing: The Microwave

I threw out the microwave.

I want to say that plainly before explaining it, because it gets the strongest reaction when I mention it — stronger than the candles, stronger than the toothpaste, stronger even than the Teflon pans. The microwave is so embedded in modern kitchen life that removing it reads, to most people, as a kind of extremism. I understand that reaction. I had it myself, briefly, before I thought it through.

The debate around microwave radiation is genuinely contested and I am not going to resolve it here. What pushed me over the edge was not the radiation. It was the food.

Microwaving heats food by agitating water molecules from the inside out — a process structurally different from every traditional cooking method human beings have ever used. Research has shown it degrades certain vitamins and antioxidants more rapidly than conventional cooking. More significantly, it destroys the living bacterial cultures in fermented foods. Microwaved bone broth is bone broth with its most delicate compounds altered. Microwaved sourdough is bread with its living cultures dead. Everything we were carefully building in those foods, undone in ninety seconds for the sake of convenience.

The microwave left. And in the space where it had been — that counter space occupied for years by an appliance designed to reheat processed food in ninety seconds — I put the tinctures. The dried herbs. The electric kettle.

The Bathroom: Personal Care and the Skin Barrier

The skin is not a wall. It is a membrane — selectively permeable, constantly absorbing what it contacts. A 2004 study by the Environmental Working Group found that the average American woman applies 168 unique chemical ingredients to her body every day through personal care products. Many have never been tested for safety in humans. The FDA does not require pre-market safety testing for cosmetic ingredients.

The soaps changed. The shampoo changed. The lotion changed. I looked for products with short ingredient lists, recognizable components, and no synthetic fragrance — because fragrance, in a personal care product, is a legal black box containing hundreds of undisclosed chemicals none of which the manufacturer is required to reveal.

And then the toothpaste. Sodium lauryl sulfate. Artificial sweeteners. Synthetic dyes. In many brands, triclosan, an antibacterial compound that disrupts thyroid function and has been found in human breast milk. We put this in our mouths twice a day. My daughters put this in their mouths twice a day.

I went completely nuts. I replaced the toothpaste. I replaced everything. And I want to be clear: I am not nuts. I was logical. I followed the same reasoning all the way to its conclusion, in every room, on every shelf, for every person in this house.

The Laundry Room

Conventional laundry detergents and fabric softeners are among the most chemically complex products in the average household, and among the least scrutinized — because we think of them as cleaning agents rather than as things we wear against our skin for sixteen hours a day. Fabric softener coats fibers with lubricating compounds associated with respiratory irritation. Dryer sheets release these as heated gases directly into the air you breathe while folding laundry.

We switched to fragrance-free, plant-based detergent. We eliminated fabric softener. The clothes are clean. Nobody is breathing synthetic musk compounds while folding laundry. The standard I applied to everything: would I be comfortable if I fully understood what this was doing inside our bodies? If the answer was no, it went.

What Happened to All of Us

I want to tell you what I watched happen over the months that followed — not just to Dave, whose recovery is the center of this book, but to my daughters, who were not sick, who did not have a diagnosis, who were simply teenagers living in a house that was being rebuilt around different principles.

They looked less drained. That is the most honest way I can describe it. The blah — that low-grade flatness that I had accepted as just how teenagers are, just how mornings work, just how it feels to be young in a body that is fed processed food and breathing synthetic air — the blah lifted. Their eyes got clearer. They were more present. More themselves. More alive in a way that I had not realized they had been slightly less alive before, because it had been the baseline for so long.

Fewer colds. Better sleep. Clearer skin. Improved digestion. Better focus at school. These are not small things in a teenager's life. These are the things that determine how a young person experiences their own body — whether it feels like something that works for them or something they are perpetually fighting.

43

They resisted at first. Of course they did. They are teenagers. Resistance is the job. But biology is more persuasive than any argument I could have made, and over time the evidence was written all over them in ways they could not ignore even if they wanted to.

And then one afternoon I sent them down the canned goods aisle while I went a different direction. I came back to find them standing in front of the crushed tomatoes, picking up one can after another, reading the labels, putting them back. Looking for the one with nothing in it but tomatoes. No citric acid derived from aspergillus niger — black mold, for anyone who has not yet had the pleasure of reading a tomato can label. Just tomatoes.

They found it. They brought it to the cart without saying a word about it.

I did not teach them that in a lesson. I did not make them read labels or explain aspergillus niger or assign them homework about the food supply. They absorbed it the way children absorb everything that actually matters — by living inside it long enough that it became their own.

There is a joke now. It started not long after Dave came home and the food had changed and we were all living inside the new version of this house together. We would drive past a fast food restaurant — one of the ones that had been a regular stop before all of this — and one of the girls would say, completely deadpan: can we get something to eat?

And Dave would say: what does your mother say?

And the girls — together, or separately, or all three of them at once including Dave — would say: that's poison.

Every single time. Windows down, driving past the drive-through, three voices and sometimes four delivering the punchline of a joke that is also, underneath the laughter, entirely true.

I set out to heal Dave. I did not set out to heal my whole family. But that is what happened, gradually and without announcement, in the months and years that followed — in the kitchen and the pantry and the grocery store aisle and every car ride past a fast food restaurant where someone asks the question and everyone already knows the answer.

That is not a side effect of this protocol. That is the point of it.

Real food, clean air, honest ingredients, and the knowledge of why it matters — these do not belong only to the person who is sick. They belong to everyone sitting at the table. Everyone sleeping under the roof. Everyone breathing the air in the house you are choosing, one decision at a time, to make into a place worth healing in.

The Philosophy Behind All of It

Modern life has normalized an extraordinary level of chemical exposure. We have been told, implicitly and explicitly, that the regulatory systems protecting us are adequate, that the amounts of any individual chemical we encounter are too small to matter, that convenience is a reasonable trade for whatever minor risks might exist.

What I will tell you is what I learned watching Dave's body try to recover, and watching my daughters thrive in ways I had not expected: the body has a finite capacity to process what it is asked to process. That capacity is called the toxic load. When the toxic load exceeds the body's processing capacity — not dramatically, not all at once, but cumulatively, over years — the result is a system perpetually slightly overwhelmed. Perpetually slightly inflamed. Perpetually slightly behind.

> *Chronic illness is increasingly understood not as the result of any single cause but as the accumulated consequence of a body that has been carrying too much for too long.*

That is what I saw happen with Dave. And with my daughters. And, quietly, with me.

Slowly, over months, as the herbs did their work and the food changed and the air got cleaner and the products on every shelf got simpler — all of our bodies began to find their way back to themselves. Not in a straight line. Not without hard days. But consistently, unmistakably, in the direction of more.

I do not think the herbs alone did that. I do not think the food alone did that. I think it was the totality of the decision — the commitment to reducing every unnecessary burden on bodies that were working as hard as they could — that created the conditions for healing to happen. For all of us.

That decision is available to anyone. It does not require a large budget or a diagnosis or a crisis dramatic enough to force the question. It just requires a willingness to look at what you have normalized, and to ask, very simply: does this need to be here?

Start with the pantry. Or the candles. Or the toothpaste. Or the microwave. Start somewhere. The body will notice. And so, eventually, will everyone else sitting at your table.

A Practical Guide: Where to Start

If you are reading this chapter and feeling overwhelmed — I hear you. I did not do all of this in a day. Here is the order I would recommend, based on where the highest exposures and highest impacts tend to be:

✓ First: The food. Clear the processed items. Find a local farm for meat. Switch to organic produce for the Environmental Working Group's Dirty Dozen at minimum. This is the highest-leverage change you can make.

✓ Second: The cooking. Replace non-stick cookware with cast iron or stainless steel. Switch plastic food storage to glass. Throw out the microwave if you are ready — or at minimum, stop using it for anything fermented, living, or nutritionally valuable.

✓ Third: The air. Remove conventional candles and synthetic air fresheners. Open windows. Let the house breathe real air.

✓ Fourth: The personal care. Use the Environmental Working Group's Skin Deep database to check your current products. Replace the highest-scoring items first. Look for short ingredient lists and no synthetic fragrance.

✓ Fifth: The laundry. Switch to fragrance-free, plant-based detergent. Eliminate fabric softener and dryer sheets.

✓ Sixth: Everything else. The toothpaste. The cleaning products. The things you stopped questioning because you have always used them. Question them now.

You do not have to do this all at once. You just have to start. And once you start — once you clear one shelf and feel the difference of a home working with your body rather than against it — the next shelf becomes easier.

Dave's recovery happened in a house that was being rebuilt around him, one decision at a time. So did my daughters'. So did mine. That is not a metaphor. It is the most literal thing I can tell you about how healing actually works.

The house is the protocol. Make it one worth healing in.

Chapter Four: Root Causes

The Question Nobody Wanted to Answer

I want to tell you about the head tilt.

You may know the one I mean. It is a very specific gesture — a slight inclination of the head, a brief softening of the expression that is almost kind, almost patient, almost respectful. It is the look a doctor gives you when you have said something they have already decided is not worth taking seriously. It is the look that says: here we go. Someone who has been on the internet.

I received that look when I brought up parasites.

Not in a frightened way, not with self-diagnosis in hand, not demanding a specific treatment. I brought it up as a question — a genuine, researched, carefully considered question about whether a body that had been through six months of broad-spectrum antibiotics, profound immune suppression, and the complete devastation of its microbial ecosystem might be hospitable to organisms that a healthy immune system would have kept in check. I had read. I had thought about it carefully. I had connected symptoms to a plausible mechanism and I was asking whether that mechanism deserved investigation.

The head tilt told me everything I needed to know about how that question was being received. Just because I had not gone to medical school, my research did not matter. My observations did not matter. My questions did not matter. I was irrelevant — a layperson who had clearly just typed something into a search engine and was now presenting the output as though it constituted medical insight.

> *So I stopped bringing it up. I did not argue. I did not try to convince anyone. I took my question, and my research, and my observations about my husband's body, and I brought them somewhere else entirely. I brought them to the herbs. I built the protocol myself. And I watched what happened.*

This chapter is for everyone who has ever received the head tilt. For everyone whose question was met with polite dismissal and who walked out of a doctor's office feeling not just unheard but somehow foolish for having asked. For everyone who went home and kept researching anyway, quietly, because the question did not go away just because someone with a medical degree had declined to engage with it.

Your questions matter. Your observations about your own body — and the bodies of the people you love — matter. The absence of a credential does not make a question less valid. It makes it less convenient. Those are not the same thing.

What the Research Actually Says

Let us begin with what is simply, documentably, unremarkably true: parasitic infections are far more common in the industrialized world than most people — including most physicians — currently acknowledge.

The Centers for Disease Control and Prevention estimates that millions of Americans are infected with parasites at any given time, with the majority of cases going undiagnosed because they are either asymptomatic in people with intact immune systems, or because the symptoms they produce — digestive irregularity, fatigue, skin issues, cognitive fog, sugar cravings — are non-specific enough to be attributed to a dozen other causes before parasitic infection is considered.

Toxoplasma gondii, estimated to infect between 11 and 40 percent of the American population depending on the study cited. Blastocystis hominis, present in up to 20 percent of the population in some surveys. Giardia lamblia, the most commonly identified intestinal parasite in the United States, infecting an estimated 1.2 million Americans annually. Pinworms, affecting an estimated 40 million Americans — the most common parasitic infection in the country, so normalized it barely registers as a medical concern despite being, by definition, parasitic.

These numbers are not from alternative medicine websites. They are from the CDC. They describe a population in which parasitic organisms are a routine biological reality — managed, in people with healthy immune systems, by the immune surveillance and microbial competition that keeps opportunistic organisms in their place.

Now remove that immune surveillance. Spend six months in an ICU on broad-spectrum antibiotics that destroy the microbial ecosystem responsible for competitive exclusion of parasitic organisms. Add the immune suppression of sedation, critical illness, and the medications required to manage it. Add the profound depletion of the micronutrients — zinc, vitamin A, vitamin D — that the immune system requires to identify and respond to parasitic threats.

What you have is not a theoretical risk. What you have is a body that has lost, temporarily but profoundly, the biological systems that keep parasitic organisms in check. The question is not whether a post-ICU patient might be more susceptible to parasitic overgrowth than a healthy person. The question — the one I asked and that received the head tilt — is simply whether that susceptibility deserves investigation.

I still believe it deserves investigation. I believe it more now than I did when I first asked the question, because I have read

The Symptoms That Led Me There

The symptoms that made me take the parasite question seriously were not exotic. They were not dramatic. They were the kind of symptoms that get a shrug in a follow-up appointment and a note in the chart that says "patient reports ongoing fatigue and digestive complaints, likely post-viral."

Digestive symptoms — the bloating, the irregularity, the discomfort that was not severe enough to constitute an emergency but was persistent enough to constitute a pattern. A gut that had been through six months of tube feeding and antibiotic devastation and was not finding its equilibrium despite the herbal digestive support, the bone broth, the sourdough, the careful rebuilding of the diet.

Skin issues that appeared without clear cause and did not respond consistently to topical treatment. The skin is the body's largest organ of elimination, and when the gut is carrying a burden it cannot process through normal channels, the skin often becomes an auxiliary elimination route — producing symptoms that look like dermatological conditions but are, at root, digestive ones.

And the cognitive fog. The brain that was not quite working the way it had before — which I had attributed entirely to post-ICU cognitive impairment and the neuroinflammatory effects of critical illness. Both of those explanations are real and valid. But parasitic organisms, particularly those with the ability to cross the gut-brain axis or produce compounds that affect neurological function, are also documented contributors to cognitive symptoms in ways that are underappreciated in conventional medicine.

Three symptom categories. Three separate specialists, potentially, in a conventional care model. One possible common root that nobody in the conventional system was willing to discuss. That is what sent me to the research. That is what made the question impossible to put down.

Why the Compromised Body Is Different

Here is the argument I could not get anyone to engage with, stated as plainly as I know how to state it.

A healthy person with an intact microbiome and a functioning immune system lives with parasitic organisms in a state of managed equilibrium. The immune system identifies them. The gut microbiome competes with them for resources. The intestinal motility clears them before they can establish. The barrier function of the gut lining prevents translocation. This is not the absence of parasitic organisms — it is the biological management of them, happening constantly and invisibly in the bodies of people who feel fine.

Strip those management systems away — through six months of broad-spectrum antibiotics, through immune suppression, through the devastation of the intestinal lining that tube feeding and pharmaceutical exposure produce, through the micronutrient depletion that critical illness generates faster than nutrition can replace — and the equilibrium breaks down. The organisms that were being held in check are no longer being held in check. The environment that was inhospitable has become hospitable. The body that was managing has lost the tools it was managing with.

This is basic microbiology. It is not controversial. It is the same logic that makes physicians vigilant about opportunistic infections in immunocompromised patients — Pneumocystis pneumonia in HIV patients, Candida overgrowth in patients on long-term antibiotics, CMV reactivation in transplant recipients. The principle that a compromised immune system loses the capacity to manage organisms it previously controlled is accepted, standard, uncontroversial medicine.

The question I was asking is simply the extension of that accepted principle to parasitic organisms specifically. If we accept that the immunocompromised body is more susceptible to opportunistic bacterial and fungal infections — and we do, without question — why would parasitic organisms be uniquely exempt from that same susceptibility?

I do not have a satisfying answer to that question. I have only the head tilt I received when I asked it. Make of that what you will.

The Protocol — Four Herbs and a Handful of Seeds

I want to be precise about what I did, because precision matters in a chapter like this one and because I am not going to tell you to do what I did. I am going to tell you what I did, why I did it, what the research behind each component shows, and what I observed. The rest is your conversation to have — with a qualified practitioner you trust, with your own research, with your own body.

The protocol we used consists of four herbs and one food. Black Walnut hull. Wormwood. Garlic. Clove. And raw pumpkin seeds. Each one addresses parasitic organisms through a different mechanism. Together they cover a broader range of parasitic life stages and species than any single agent can address alone. That comprehensiveness is the logic of the combination — and it is a combination that has appeared in traditional antiparasitic medicine across multiple cultures for centuries, long before any of us had words like mechanism of action or bioactive compound.

We ran it in cycles — on and off over time — rather than as a single defined course. This matters because parasite life cycles mean that a single course of any antiparasitic treatment may address adults but miss eggs and larvae that mature after the treatment ends. Cycling, with rest periods between, accounts for those life cycles and creates the sustained, repeated unfavorable environment that a one-time intervention cannot.

Both of us did it — Dave and I. Not because I was certain I had a parasitic burden. But because the logic of a shared household, shared meals, and a shared history of stress-mediated immune compromise made the question relevant for both of us. And because the herbs involved are safe, well-studied, and used correctly present no meaningful risk to a healthy adult.

Black Walnut Hull

Juglans nigra

The hull of the black walnut — the green outer casing of the nut, harvested before it blackens — contains juglone, a naphthalene derivative with documented antiparasitic, antifungal, and antibacterial properties. Juglone creates an inhospitable environment for a wide range of parasitic organisms by interfering with their cellular energy production — a mechanism that affects parasitic organisms far more than it affects human cells, because of differences in metabolic pathway dependence between parasitic and mammalian biology.

Black Walnut hull has been used in traditional medicine across Native American, European, and Chinese traditions for intestinal parasites. The tannins in the hull also have astringent properties that reduce the intestinal inflammation that parasitic colonization produces and that support the restoration of healthy intestinal barrier function during and after an antiparasitic protocol.

Tincture from the farm, standardized to the green hull harvested at peak juglone content. This is the preparation we use — quality and timing of harvest matter significantly for juglone content, which is why sourcing from a farm that understands the plant is not optional.

Wormwood

Wormwood is the herb that gives absinthe its name and its bitterness, and it has been used as an antiparasitic herb in virtually every culture that knew it for at least two thousand years. Its primary active compound, artemisinin, is a sesquiterpene lactone that has been the subject of serious pharmaceutical research — it is the basis of artemisinin-based combination therapies, currently the most effective pharmaceutical treatments for malaria in use worldwide.

The fact that a compound derived from Wormwood is the gold standard pharmaceutical treatment for one of the world's most significant parasitic diseases is not an argument for herbalism over medicine. It is an illustration of the principle that runs through this entire book: traditional use, accumulated over centuries of observation, is frequently pointing at real mechanisms. The research catches up eventually.

Beyond malaria specifically, artemisinin and related compounds in Wormwood have documented activity against a range of intestinal parasites including Giardia, Ascaris, and pinworms. The bitter compounds — absinthin and artabsin — stimulate bile production and digestive secretions that create an inhospitable environment for parasitic organisms in the upper digestive tract, where Black Walnut hull's primary activity is more distal.

Wormwood is a potent herb and should be used with respect. It is not for long-term continuous use — the thujone content, while low in properly prepared preparations, accumulates with extended use. Cycling is the appropriate approach, which aligns exactly with the cycling protocol we used. Tincture from the farm, where the preparation is controlled and the thujone content managed appropriately.

Clove

Syzygium aromaticum

Clove's role in the antiparasitic protocol is specific and important: it addresses parasitic eggs and larvae, the life stages that Black Walnut and Wormwood address less completely. Eugenol — the primary active compound in clove, responsible for its characteristic sharp, warm scent — has documented ovicidal activity against a range of parasitic species, disrupting the egg membranes of intestinal parasites and preventing the hatching that allows a new generation to establish.

This is why the three herbs are used together rather than separately. Black Walnut and Wormwood address adult parasitic organisms through their respective mechanisms. Clove addresses the eggs. Without all three, you address part of the life cycle while the rest continues uninterrupted. The comprehensiveness of the combination is its clinical logic.

Clove also has broad antimicrobial and antifungal properties through its eugenol content, making it useful beyond the specific antiparasitic application for the general gut environment restoration that is the larger goal of this protocol. A gut that is simultaneously clearing parasitic organisms, rebalancing its microbial ecosystem, and restoring its barrier function benefits from the breadth of clove's antimicrobial coverage.

Garlic

Allium sativum — See Full Profile

Garlic's role in the antiparasitic protocol draws on the same allicin activity covered in its full herb profile earlier in this reference. Allicin's disruption of sulfhydryl-containing enzymes essential to parasitic metabolism creates a direct hostile environment for a range of intestinal parasites, and its broad antimicrobial action addresses the bacterial overgrowth that often coexists with and supports parasitic colonization.

In the protocol context, garlic serves as both the fourth antiparasitic agent and the daily food-level exposure that maintains a baseline inhospitable environment between protocol cycles. The tincture during active cycling. The daily cooking with properly prepared garlic — crushed, rested, then cooked — as the sustained background protocol that never stops. This dual application is what distinguishes garlic from the other three herbs in this combination: it is simultaneously a medicine and a food, and both applications serve the same end.

Raw Pumpkin Seeds

Cucurbita pepo — The Overlooked Fifth Agent

Raw pumpkin seeds are not an herb. They are food — which is precisely why they belong in this chapter alongside the herbs, and why they deserve more attention than they typically receive in the antiparasitic conversation.

Cucurbitacin — a tetracyclic triterpene compound found in the seeds of Cucurbita species — has documented antiparasitic activity through a mechanism that is elegantly different from every other agent in this protocol: it paralyzes the nervous system of intestinal worms, causing them to release their grip on the intestinal wall so that normal peristalsis can carry them out of the body. No cellular toxicity. No disruption of human metabolic pathways. A compound that is selectively disruptive to parasitic nervous systems in a way that does not affect mammalian neurology.

Pumpkin seeds have been used as an antiparasitic food across Central America, Africa, Asia, and Europe for centuries — given to children for pinworms, used by traditional healers for intestinal worms of multiple species, employed in folk medicine traditions that had no contact with each other but independently reached the same conclusion about the same seed.

Raw is essential. The cucurbitacin content is reduced by roasting. Whole, raw, organic pumpkin seeds — a handful daily during active protocol cycles, eaten as a food rather than taken as a supplement. This is medicine that costs nothing, requires no prescription, produces no side effects, and has been working in human digestive systems for as long as humans have been eating pumpkins.

It is also the detail that most practitioners skip entirely. I include it because it is what we used, because the research supports it, and because a book about healing that omits the simplest, most accessible tools in favor of the more exotic ones is a book that has lost sight of its purpose.

What We Observed

I am a witness in this book, not a clinician. I cannot tell you what the protocol did. I can tell you what I observed, and I can be precise about the limits of that observation.

Over the course of the cycling protocol — run over months, with rest periods between courses, in both Dave and myself — the digestive symptoms that had persisted despite the broader herbal protocol and the dietary overhaul began to shift. The bloating that had been a consistent background feature became intermittent, then occasional, then largely absent. The irregularity resolved into a pattern that felt, for the first time since he came home, like a gut that had found its rhythm.

The skin issues that had appeared without clear cause and resisted topical treatment improved. Not immediately, not linearly, but over the weeks and months of the protocol in a way that correlated with nothing else we had changed.

The cognitive fog — the hardest symptom to attribute with any confidence, because so many things affect cognitive function and because Dave's post-ICU brain had multiple legitimate explanations for impairment — continued its gradual improvement during the period of the protocol. I cannot say the protocol caused that improvement. I can say the improvement happened and the protocol was running.

How to Find a Practitioner Who Will Listen

The dismissal I received from conventional physicians is not universal. There are practitioners — integrative medicine physicians, naturopathic doctors, functional medicine practitioners — who bring the rigor of medical training to questions that conventional medicine has not yet decided to take seriously. Who will order a comprehensive stool analysis. Who will consider parasitic burden as a genuine clinical question rather than an internet-generated anxiety. Who will engage with a patient who has done research as a collaborator rather than a problem.

Finding those practitioners is worth the effort. They exist. They are not on every corner and they are not always covered by standard insurance, which is its own injustice in a healthcare system that claims to prioritize prevention. But they are there, and a patient who arrives with genuine observations, genuine research, and genuine questions about root causes deserves a practitioner who will meet them there.

If you cannot find one immediately, the functional medicine and integrative medicine directories — the Institute for Functional Medicine physician finder, the American Association of Naturopathic Physicians directory — are reasonable starting points. A practitioner willing to order a GI-MAP or comprehensive digestive stool analysis is already demonstrating a different level of engagement with the gut as a system than the standard of care typically provides.

You deserve a practitioner who treats your questions as data rather than noise. Do not stop looking until you find one.

The Antiparasitic Protocol — Practical Guidance

What follows is the protocol we used, described precisely and without embellishment. I am not prescribing this for you. I am describing what we did so that you have accurate information when you have the conversation with a qualified practitioner who is willing to engage with it seriously.

The Four-Herb Tincture Protocol

All four herb tinctures sourced from the farm — quality and sourcing are non-negotiable for this protocol. Black Walnut hull must be from green hulls harvested at peak juglone content. Wormwood must be properly prepared to appropriate thujone levels. Clove and Garlic tinctures from whole, properly harvested plant material.

Suggested Protocol — Cycling Approach:

Week 1–2: Black Walnut hull tincture, 1–2 ml three times daily. Wormwood tincture, 1 ml twice daily. Clove tincture, 1 ml twice daily. Garlic tincture, 1–2 ml twice daily.

Week 3–4: Rest period. Continue garlic in food daily. Continue raw pumpkin seeds daily.

Repeat cycle 2–3 times over 2–3 months to address multiple parasite life cycles.

During active protocol: increase water intake significantly to support elimination. Add Burdock Root and Milk Thistle to support the liver's processing of die-off compounds.

Raw Pumpkin Seeds — Daily During Protocol:

1–2 handfuls of raw, organic pumpkin seeds daily.

Eaten raw — do not roast, as heat reduces cucurbitacin content.

Can be eaten plain, added to salads, blended into smoothies.

Continue through rest periods as a maintenance food.

Important Notes:

- Not for use during pregnancy or while breastfeeding.
- Wormwood is not for long-term continuous use — cycling is essential.
- Support liver function throughout with Milk Thistle and Burdock Root tinctures.
- Some people experience a temporary worsening of symptoms during the first days of the protocol — known as a Herxheimer or die-off reaction as parasitic organisms are cleared. This typically resolves within a few days. If severe, reduce doses and consult a practitioner.
- Do not run this protocol without discussing it with a practitioner if managing serious health conditions or taking pharmaceutical medications.

I want to close this chapter where I opened it — with the question that received the head tilt, and with what I want to say to the doctor who gave it to me.

I understand that you see patients who have read things on the internet and arrived at conclusions that are not supported by evidence. I understand that this is a genuine and frustrating part of your work. I understand that the signal-to-noise ratio of patient-generated research varies enormously, and that sorting through it takes time you may not have.

But here is what I need you to understand: I was not noise. I was a woman who had spent six months in a medical system that saved my husband's life and then handed him back to me with twelve pages of discharge instructions and no roadmap for what came next. I had filled the gap the only way I knew how — by reading, by questioning, by paying closer attention to his body than any monitor could. My question was not the product of a search engine. It was the product of months of sustained, careful observation by the person who knew him best.

I did not need you to agree with me. I needed you to engage with me. There is a difference.

I stopped bringing it up. I did not stop being right to ask.

To every reader who has received their own version of the head tilt — for this question or for any other question that deserved better than dismissal: your questions are data. Your observations about your own body are data. The absence of a medical degree does not make them less true. It makes them less legible to a system that has decided it only reads certain languages.

Learn enough to translate. Find practitioners who already speak yours. And do not let anyone's head tilt be the last word on a question that your body is still asking.

A Note Before You Begin

I want to tell you something before you turn the first page of this reference section, because I think it matters and because no one told me when I was starting out.

I am not a master herbalist. I did not apprentice with a healer in the mountains of Appalachia or study at a formal botanical school. What I am is a woman who needed to learn, and who learned by doing — by reading everything I could find, by asking questions of people who knew more than I did, by making mistakes and correcting them, and by watching, over time, what actually helped.

Some of the herbs in this section I grow myself. Mullein, for instance, grows in my yard without any encouragement from me — a tall, silver-green spike appearing each summer in the disturbed soil at the edge of the property, as though it knows it is needed. I harvest its leaves, dry them, and make tea. It costs nothing. It requires almost no skill. It is one of the most powerful lung herbs on earth, and it may already be growing at the edge of yours.

> *But I will not pretend that I make everything myself. I do not. My tinctures — the*

Here is what I have come to believe about sourcing: the quality of what goes into a preparation determines the quality of what you get out of it. A tincture made from herbs grown in depleted soil, harvested at the wrong time, extracted with cheap alcohol, and sitting in a warehouse for eighteen months before it reaches your door is not the same thing as a tincture made by a family who knows their land, harvests by hand at peak potency, and packs their bottles the same week they are ordered.

The difference is not subtle. It is the difference between medicine and the idea of medicine.

This is why, throughout this book, I will encourage you to grow what you can, make what you are able, and buy the rest from people you can look in the eye — or at minimum, whose farm you could visit if you wanted to. Small, organic, family-run herb farms are not a luxury. They are a standard. And they are worth every penny of the price difference.

How to Use This Reference

The herb profiles that follow are organized alphabetically — so if you know what you are looking for, you can find it directly. But the book also includes two additional indexes at the back: one organized by body system, and one organized by ailment. If you are not sure which herb to reach for, start there. Tell the index what is happening in the body, and let it point you toward the plants.

Each profile includes the herb's Latin name, its primary traditional and documented uses, the science behind its active compounds, its connection to Dave's specific recovery where relevant, and at least one recipe. Most profiles include both a tea and a tincture preparation, because different situations call for different delivery methods — and I want you to have options.

A few things I ask you to keep in mind as you read:

These profiles are written for educational purposes. They are not a prescription, a diagnosis, or a replacement for the relationship between you and your healthcare provider. If you are managing a serious illness, taking pharmaceuticals, or caring for someone who is, please involve a qualified practitioner — ideally one who is fluent in both conventional medicine and botanical healing. They exist, and they are worth finding.

Herbs are not inert. They are bioactive, which means they can interact with medications, affect lab results, and contraindicate certain conditions. I note the most significant cautions in each profile, but I am not a clinician and this list is not exhaustive. Do your research. Ask your doctor. And when in doubt, start low and go slow.

With that said — do not let caution become paralysis. Human beings have been using these plants safely for thousands of years. The risks, for most people in most circumstances, are modest. The potential benefits, as Dave's story suggests, are anything but.

On Quality: What to Look For

Whether you are buying dried herbs, tinctures, salves, or infused oils, here is what separates a product worth your trust from one that is not:

✓ Organic or beyond organic — meaning grown without synthetic pesticides, herbicides, or chemical fertilizers. Certified organic is the standard, but many small farms practice organic methods without the expensive certification. Ask.

✓ Small batch — meaning the herbs were processed in quantities small enough that someone was paying attention to each one. Industrial herb processing is not the same as hand-harvested, hand-packed preparation.

✓ Harvested at peak potency — meaning the farmer knows when each plant is at its most medicinally active and harvests accordingly. Roots in autumn, when energy has returned underground. Flowers at full bloom. Leaves before the plant goes to seed.

✓ Transparent about sourcing — meaning the farm can tell you where every ingredient comes from. If they grow it themselves, even better. If they source from other farms, those should be farms they know and trust.

✓ Freshly made — meaning tinctures are not sitting in a warehouse for years before reaching you. Ask about production dates. A good farm will tell you.

✓ Made by people who use what they make — meaning this is not a business built on a trend. The best herbalists I have encountered are people who have been living with these plants for decades, who grow them in their gardens and take them in their own kitchens and give them to their own families.

A Farm Worth Knowing

I want to mention, with their permission, the farm where I source most of my tinctures, dried herbs, salves, and infused oils. I found them in the early months of Dave's recovery, when I knew what I needed but had not yet found someone I trusted to make it. What I found was a family operation run by people who treat their plants the way I treat my patients — with attention, with respect, and with the understanding that what you put in determines what you get out.

I have been buying from them ever since. I do not receive anything in return for mentioning them. I mention them because this book is about telling the truth, and the truth is that access to high-quality herbal preparations changed Dave's recovery — and that access came through them.

If you are not able to source from a small farm — whether for reasons of geography, budget, or availability — the following general guidance will help you evaluate what is available to you. Look for the markers listed above. Read ingredient labels carefully. Choose whole herb preparations over proprietary blends where possible, so you know exactly what you are getting. And whenever you can, buy from a human being rather than an algorithm.

On Making Your Own

If you want to make your own preparations — and I hope some of you do, because there is something deeply satisfying about it — each herb profile in this section includes the herb's background, the science behind it, how it was used in Dave's recovery, and personal notes on sourcing and use.

Start with tea. Tea is forgiving and immediate and requires almost no investment. A jar of dried Mullein leaf costs a few dollars. Boiling water is free. If you want to go further, a basic tincture requires a mason jar, your herb of choice, and a bottle of vodka. That is genuinely all.

The recipes in this book are written the way I learned them — from Rosemary Gladstar's foundational work, from Susun Weed, from the accumulated wisdom of herbalists who have been teaching people to make their own medicine for decades. Where I have adapted or simplified, I say so. Where I follow tradition, I cite it.

One final thing. When you make something with your own hands — when you measure and mix and label and wait — you are participating in something that goes back as far as human beings have been sick and have wanted to get better. Every kitchen apothecary in history started exactly where you are starting: with a plant, some water, and the decision to try.

That decision is not small. It is, in fact, the whole point.

The herb profiles begin on the following page, starting with Burdock Root. The complete A-Z reference, body systems index, and ailment index follow in sequence.

Burdock Root

There is a plant that most of us have cursed at one time or another without knowing its name. Its seed heads — the round, hooked burrs that attach themselves to clothing and animal fur with remarkable tenacity — are the botanical inspiration for Velcro. George de Mestral, the Swiss engineer who invented the fastening system in 1941, reportedly got the idea after pulling Burdock burrs from his dog's coat and examining them under a microscope.

The plant behind those burrs is one of the most powerful detoxifying herbs in the traditional pharmacopoeia of both East and West. Burdock Root has been used in Traditional Chinese Medicine for more than two thousand years, where it is known as Niubang and prescribed for heat conditions, toxic accumulation, and inflammation. In European herbalism it appears in texts going back to the medieval period, consistently described as a blood purifier and liver tonic. In Japan, the root is eaten as a vegetable — called gobo — and has been a staple of the diet for centuries, valued as much for its health properties as its flavor.

A plant that three entirely independent medical traditions — Chinese, European, and Japanese — reached for independently, for overlapping reasons, over overlapping centuries, is worth paying very close attention to.

What those traditions understood empirically, modern phytochemistry has begun to explain mechanically. Burdock Root contains an impressive concentration of inulin — a prebiotic fiber that feeds beneficial gut bacteria and supports the microbiome that prolonged antibiotic use devastates. It contains arctiin and arctigenin, lignans with documented anti-inflammatory, antioxidant, and antimicrobial properties. It contains polyacetylenes with demonstrated antibacterial activity. And it contains a range of bitter compounds that stimulate bile production in the liver and gallbladder, supporting the body's primary detoxification organ in doing its work more efficiently.

> *After six months of antibiotics, antivirals, immunosuppressants, sedatives, and pain medications — Dave's liver was not simply tired. It had been running a marathon in full armor for half a year. Burdock Root was the first thing I reached for on its behalf.*

But the liver story is only part of what makes Burdock Root remarkable. The other part — the part that conventional medicine tends to skip over entirely — is its relationship to the lymphatic system and the skin.

The lymphatic system is the body's secondary circulatory network, responsible for collecting cellular waste, transporting immune cells, and filtering pathogens through the lymph nodes before returning fluid to the bloodstream. When the liver is overburdened and cannot process the toxic load efficiently, the lymphatic system compensates — and when the lymphatic system is itself overwhelmed, the skin becomes the overflow valve. This is why prolonged illness, pharmaceutical burden, and systemic inflammation so often manifest visibly in the skin: rashes, breakouts, dullness, unusual textures.

Burdock Root supports all three systems simultaneously — liver, lymph, and skin — which is why herbalists have historically described it as a blood purifier. That phrase sounds archaic, but it is pointing at something real: a plant that helps the body's filtration systems do their jobs, so that what circulates through the body is cleaner than what went in.

In his comprehensive reference Medical Herbalism: The Science and Practice of Herbal Medicine, clinical herbalist David Hoffmann describes Burdock as "one of the most reliable herbs for treating skin conditions that result from systemic toxicity," and notes its particular value in chronic conditions where the elimination organs — liver, kidneys, skin, lymph — need sustained, gentle support rather than acute intervention.

Sustained and gentle is exactly right. Burdock Root is not a dramatic herb. It does not act fast and forcefully the way some plants do. It works slowly, steadily, over weeks and months, gradually reducing the toxic burden on systems that have been carrying too much for too long. For Dave's recovery — which was measured not in days but in seasons — that pace was exactly what was needed.

This raises a question that I think about often: why does conventional medicine so rarely address what prolonged pharmaceutical treatment does to the liver, the gut, and the lymphatic system? The medications that saved Dave's life also left a significant biological debt. That debt did not appear on his discharge paperwork. It appeared in his body, slowly, over the months that followed. Burdock Root was part of how we paid it back.

A Word on Parasites

Burdock Root has a long traditional history of use as an antiparasitic — one of the quieter aspects of its profile that deserves more attention than it typically receives.

The subject of parasites in human health is one that mainstream Western medicine has historically underestimated, at least in the context of developed nations. The assumption has long been that parasitic infection is primarily a concern in tropical or developing regions. Increasingly, researchers and integrative practitioners are questioning that assumption. A 2019 review in the journal Parasitology Research noted that intestinal parasitic infections are significantly more prevalent in industrialized nations than standard diagnostic practice tends to detect — in part because routine testing looks for a narrow range of organisms and misses many others entirely.

This matters for a book rooted in root causes. If the question is not merely "what are the symptoms?" but "why is the body behaving this way?" — then parasitic load is a variable that belongs in the conversation. Chronic fatigue, digestive irregularity, skin conditions, immune dysregulation, and inflammatory patterns that resist conventional treatment are all associated in the integrative literature with undetected parasitic burden.

Burdock Root's bitter compounds and polyacetylenes create an environment in the gut that is less hospitable to parasitic organisms, while simultaneously supporting the beneficial bacteria that are the gut's first line of defense. It is not the most

aggressive antiparasitic herb in the botanical world —
that distinction belongs to others, which we will discuss
in their own profiles — but it is a foundational support,
the kind of herb that makes the terrain of the body less
welcoming to what should not be there.

We will address the parasite question in much
greater depth in a dedicated chapter later in this book.
For now, know that Burdock Root belongs in any
protocol that takes seriously the question of what the
body might be hosting without your knowledge or
consent.

*Burdock Root came in alongside Milk Thistle as part of
a liver and lymphatic support protocol. We used a
tincture from the farm — started slowly, one
preparation at a time, watching how the body
responded.*

*A note for the reader managing post-hospitalization
recovery, post-COVID sequelae, or any condition
involving prolonged pharmaceutical treatment:
Burdock Root and Milk Thistle together form what I
think of as the foundation of a recovery protocol. The
liver cannot heal what it cannot process. Give it what it
needs to do its job, and the rest of the body begins to
follow.*

That sense, when it comes, is unmistakable. And it is
worth the wait.

Body Systems: Liver & Gallbladder | Lymphatic | Digestive | Skin

Ailments: Post-Pharmaceutical Recovery, Skin Conditions, Lymphatic Congestion, Digestive Sluggishness, Parasitic Support

Chamomile

Matricaria chamomilla | The Great Calmer

If there is one herb that almost every person on earth has encountered in some form — in a tea bag at a hotel, in a bedtime blend from a pharmacy shelf, in a grandmother's kitchen — it is this one. Chamomile is so familiar that we have nearly stopped seeing it. And that familiarity, as is so often the case with things hiding in plain sight, has caused us to dramatically underestimate what it is capable of.

Let us start by saying this clearly: Chamomile is not a placebo. It is not the botanical equivalent of a warm bath and a kind word, though it will give you something of both. It is a pharmacologically active plant whose compounds have been the subject of serious scientific investigation for decades, with a body of research substantial enough to fill several volumes. The fact that it also happens to be gentle, widely available, and deeply pleasant to drink is not a mark against it. That is simply what good medicine sometimes looks like.

The ancient Egyptians considered Chamomile so sacred they dedicated it to the sun god Ra and used it in the embalming process. The Romans used it as incense and as medicine. The Anglo-Saxons listed it as one of nine sacred herbs. In the folk medicine of virtually every European culture, it was the first thing reached for when a child could not sleep, when a stomach was in revolt, when anxiety had taken up residence in the chest and would not leave.

Two thousand years of reaching for the same flower when the nervous system needs help is a data set worth taking seriously.

The primary active compounds in Chamomile are apigenin — a flavonoid that binds to benzodiazepine receptors in the brain, the same receptors targeted by anti-anxiety medications like Valium — and alpha-bisabolol, a terpenoid with potent anti-inflammatory, antimicrobial, and antispasmodic properties. The essential oil also contains chamazulene, which gives German Chamomile its characteristic deep blue color when distilled and contributes significantly to its anti-inflammatory activity.

The research on Chamomile and anxiety is not ambiguous. It has been tested in clinical trials against placebo and it works — meaningfully, measurably, with a safety profile that puts most pharmaceutical alternatives to shame. That is not an opinion. That is what the studies show.

> *For Dave, coming home with the fractured sleep, the hypervigilance, and the low hum of anxiety that follows prolonged critical*

Post-Intensive Care Syndrome — PICS — includes a psychological dimension that is well documented and rarely adequately addressed at discharge. Studies suggest that between 30 and 50 percent of MICU survivors experience clinically significant anxiety in the year following hospitalization, with rates of PTSD approaching those seen in combat veterans. The nervous system that has spent months in a state of managed crisis does not simply switch off when the crisis ends. It remains alert, poised, scanning for the next emergency that may or may not come.

This is not weakness. This is neurobiology. The amygdala — the brain's threat-detection center — has been running on high for months. Telling it to stand down with words does not work. It has to be shown, repeatedly, through the body, that safety is real. This is where Chamomile earns its place not as an occasional comfort but as a daily practice.

Apigenin's affinity for the benzodiazepine receptor is the mechanism, but the ritual is the message. A warm cup of Chamomile in the evening, steeped slowly, drunk without screens or noise — that is a signal sent to a nervous system that has forgotten what quiet feels like. Done consistently, over weeks and months, it begins to rewrite the baseline. Not dramatically. Gently. The way all real healing happens.

Beyond anxiety and sleep, Chamomile carries a remarkable range of additional actions that made it particularly suited to Dave's recovery. Its anti-inflammatory compounds reduce systemic inflammation, which was significantly elevated after months of infection and immune response. Its antispasmodic properties ease the digestive cramping and irritable bowel symptoms that frequently accompany prolonged antibiotic use and the disrupted gut microbiome that follows. Its mild bitter compounds support digestion and liver function. It is, in the language of herbalism, what is called a trophorestorative — an herb that does not simply address a symptom but restores tone and function to a depleted system over time.

Herbalist Matthew Wood, whose book The Earthwise Herbal is one of the most thorough botanical references available to the English-language reader, describes Chamomile as the herb for "the person who is irritable, oversensitive, and exhausted — who has given too much and has nothing left." He could have been describing every MICU survivor I have ever read about. He could have been describing me.

A question worth sitting with: how many of the symptoms we treat in isolation — the insomnia, the digestive trouble, the low-grade anxiety, the inflammation that will not fully resolve — are the nervous system's way of saying it has not yet been told the emergency is over? And what would it mean to treat the nervous system first, before reaching for something more targeted?

Chamomile does not treat one thing. It treats the state that underlies many things. That is a different and, I would argue, a more sophisticated kind of medicine than we give it credit for.

For Dave, Chamomile was a clinical decision — not a comfort measure. The fractured sleep, the hypervigilance, the low hum of anxiety that follows critical illness. I used it as a tincture from the farm, combined with Lemon Balm during the worst periods. I also made it as a covered tea in the evenings — covered, always, to keep the volatile oils from escaping with the steam.

The quiet, when it comes, is real.

Body Systems: Nervous System | Digestive | Immune | Skin (topical)

Ailments: Anxiety, Insomnia, Post-ICU Recovery, Digestive Spasm, IBS, Inflammation, PTSD Support, Caregiver Burnout

Echinacea

Echinacea purpurea, E. angustifolia, E. pallida | The Innate Immune Activator

If Elderberry is the herb that intercepts a virus before it takes hold, Echinacea is the herb that wakes the immune system up to fight it. The two work differently, through different mechanisms, on different aspects of the immune response — which is exactly why we use them together, simultaneously, at the first sign of anything coming.

Echinacea is the most commercially sold herbal supplement in the United States and has been for decades. It is also one of the most misused — bought in low-quality capsule form from a pharmacy shelf, taken sporadically or incorrectly, sourced from material of unknown origin and questionable potency, and then dismissed when it fails to produce results. The conclusion people draw is that Echinacea does not work. The correct conclusion is that what they were taking was not Echinacea in any meaningful sense.

Quality, preparation, and timing are everything with this herb. A well-made tincture from whole plant material, taken at the right moment in the right dose, is a genuinely different thing from a standardized extract capsule that has been sitting on a warehouse shelf for eighteen months. I cannot say this clearly enough,

Echinacea is native to North America — one of the few major medicinal herbs in this reference that is. The Plains nations used it extensively for centuries before European settlers learned of it: for infections, for snake bites, for septic conditions, for anything involving inflammation and immune challenge. By the late nineteenth century it had become the most widely used medicinal plant in the United States, prescribed by physicians and sold by pharmacies. Then antibiotics arrived, and Echinacea was dismissed as folk medicine. What the dismissal missed is that Echinacea and antibiotics address different problems. Antibiotics target bacteria. They do nothing for viruses. Echinacea activates the immune system's own capacity to identify and respond to both.

The active compounds in Echinacea include alkamides — particularly in E. purpurea and E. angustifolia — which directly bind to cannabinoid receptors in the immune system and modulate cytokine production. They include polysaccharides that activate macrophages — the immune cells responsible for identifying and engulfing pathogens. And they include caffeic acid derivatives, including echinacoside and cichoric acid, with antioxidant and antiviral properties.

The whole family uses it. At the first sign. Every time. And in our experience — across multiple cold and flu seasons, with two daughters who are home with us and still move through the world — errands, activities, people they encounter — illnesses have been shorter, less severe, and in many cases intercepted before they fully developed.

I am not a physician and I cannot tell you that will be your experience. I can tell you it has been ours.

Species, Parts, and Why It Matters

There are three species of Echinacea used medicinally, and they are not interchangeable. E. purpurea — the most widely available and most studied — is particularly effective in above-ground preparations: the aerial parts, flowers, and fresh juice. E. angustifolia root is considered by many clinical herbalists to be the most potent species for immune activation, with a higher concentration of alkamides. E. pallida root is used primarily for its polysaccharide content.

The root and the aerial parts also have different activity profiles. Root preparations — particularly from E. angustifolia — tend to be more concentrated and longer acting. Aerial preparations from E. purpurea work faster but are shorter acting. A tincture made from a combination of species and plant parts captures the broadest range of activity.

When sourcing Echinacea, look for a farm that specifies the species and plant part used. If they cannot tell you which species and which part of the plant their tincture contains, find a different source.

The Timing Question — How Long to Use It

There is a widely repeated claim that Echinacea should not be used for more than two weeks continuously because it will "stop working" or "overstimulate" the immune system. This claim is not well supported by the clinical research and appears to have originated from a misinterpretation of early German regulatory guidance that was itself based on theoretical concern rather than clinical evidence.

The current consensus among clinical herbalists and the majority of the research literature is that Echinacea is safe for extended use, that the concern about immune overstimulation is not supported by human clinical trials, and that the most appropriate guidance is: use it actively at the onset and during illness, use it preventively during high-exposure periods, and follow your body's response.

The one genuine caution is for people with autoimmune conditions, where any immune-stimulating herb should be used under the guidance of a qualified practitioner. If you are managing an autoimmune condition, please have that conversation before using Echinacea regularly.

Dave came home with lungs that could not afford a respiratory infection. Echinacea tincture from the farm — combined always with Elderberry — was the first thing off the counter at any sign of illness, and part of the preventive protocol during cold and flu season.

Keep it on the counter. Know how to use it. Use it early. In our experience, that is the difference between a cold that lasts a week and one that never fully arrives.

Body Systems: Immune | Lymphatic | Upper Respiratory

Ailments: Cold and Flu Prevention, Viral Illness, Bacterial Infection, Immune Depletion, Post-ICU Immune Recovery, Respiratory Infection

Isatis

Isatis tinctoria / Isatis indigotica | Ban Lan Gen | The Eastern Antiviral

Most readers of this book will not recognize this herb by name. That is precisely the problem this profile is here to solve.

Isatis — known in Traditional Chinese Medicine as Ban Lan Gen, from the root, and Da Qing Ye from the leaf — has been used in Chinese medicine for over two thousand years. It appears in the Shennong Bencao Jing, one of the foundational texts of Chinese herbal medicine, classified as a cold, bitter herb indicated for heat conditions — which in the language of TCM means exactly what it sounds like: fever, acute infection, inflammation, the body in the acute phase of fighting something serious.

It is not well known in the Western herbal tradition. It is extraordinarily well known in the Eastern one. And when the SARS outbreak struck in 2003, Chinese public health authorities incorporated isatis preparations into official prevention and treatment protocols used across the country. During COVID-19, it appeared again in Chinese medical guidelines for early-stage treatment. A government medical system does not reach for a plant in a public health emergency unless that plant has two thousand years of consistent results behind it.

The active compounds in isatis include indirubin and indigo — the same pigments that give the plant its historical use as a blue dye — along with tryptanthrin, sinigrin, and a range of alkaloids and glucosinolates with documented antiviral, antibacterial, and anti-inflammatory properties. Modern research has identified isatis as active against a broad spectrum of respiratory pathogens including influenza viruses, respiratory syncytial virus, and several strains of bacteria responsible for secondary respiratory infections.

The research on Isatis is specific and consistent — documented activity against influenza virus replication, interference with viral attachment to host cells, and anti-inflammatory compounds that address the immune overreaction that makes respiratory illness dangerous. It is not a well-known herb in Western practice. That does not mean it does not work. It means fewer people have thought to study it.

The anti-inflammatory activity of isatis compounds is equally well documented, with indirubin in particular showing potent inhibition of inflammatory cytokines through pathways that overlap with those targeted by pharmaceutical anti-inflammatory agents — without, in the research literature, the gastrointestinal and cardiovascular side effects associated with those agents.

A question that occurs to me every cold and flu season: why is this herb not in every Western medicine cabinet? The research exists. The traditional record spans two millennia. The mechanism is increasingly well understood. The answer, I suspect, is the same answer that applies to Wild Lettuce and to every other effective plant that has been quietly sidelined by a medical culture organized around patentable compounds. Isatis cannot be owned. So it is not marketed. So most people have never heard of it.

You have now.

Isatis in the Context of Respiratory Recovery

For Dave, the context that made isatis relevant was specific: a man with post-ventilator lungs, an immune system in active recovery, and a respiratory tract that had been through more trauma than most bodies ever experience. In that context, the secondary bacterial infections that can follow viral respiratory illness were not a theoretical risk. They were a realistic one. Lungs that have been on a ventilator for five months do not have the same mucosal barrier integrity, the same ciliary function, the same local immune defense capacity as healthy lungs. They are more vulnerable to exactly what isatis addresses.

During the cold and flu seasons following his discharge, isatis tincture was part of the protocol specifically for any illness that involved the throat or the upper respiratory tract — the scratchy throat, the developing cough, anything that suggested the infection was heading downward. Combined with elderberry and echinacea for systemic immune support, and Mullein for the lungs themselves, it formed a respiratory illness response protocol that addressed the infection from multiple angles simultaneously.

In our experience, that layered approach — each herb doing something different, none of them redundant — is what makes the difference between an illness that resolves quickly and one that lingers and deepens. The body is not a simple system. Neither is the protocol that supports it.

A Note on Sourcing Isatis

Isatis is less widely available than elderberry or echinacea in Western herb markets, which makes sourcing from a quality farm even more important. Look for tinctures that specify the plant part used — root preparations (Ban Lan Gen) are the most widely researched and most commonly used for acute antiviral applications. Leaf preparations (Da Qing Ye) have overlapping but slightly different activity and are also legitimate.

As with all herbs in this reference: whole plant material from a trusted small farm, properly extracted, recently made. Not a capsule of unknown origin from a supplement aisle. If your source cannot tell you where the plant was grown and how the tincture was made, find a different source.

During the cold and flu seasons following Dave's discharge, Isatis tincture was part of the protocol specifically for any illness that involved the throat or the upper respiratory tract. We used it from the farm, combined with Elderberry and Echinacea.

That is not a prescription. That is a record. And the record speaks for itself.

Body Systems: Immune | Respiratory | Antiviral | Anti-inflammatory

Ailments: Throat Infection, Upper Respiratory Infection, Influenza, Viral Illness, Bacterial Respiratory Infection, Fever, Post-ICU Respiratory Recovery

Elderberry

There is a protocol in our house that has not changed since the first months of Dave's recovery, and it goes like this: at the first sign of illness — the scratchy throat, the sudden fatigue, the feeling that something is coming — the elderberry tincture comes out. The echinacea tincture comes out alongside it. And we do not wait to see how bad it gets.

We act immediately. That is the whole strategy.

I want to tell you why that strategy exists before I tell you about the herb itself, because the why is the most important part. When Dave came home from the hospital in September 2021, his lungs were not simply healing. They were fragile in a way that is difficult to overstate — tissue that had been mechanically ventilated for five months, that had survived ECMO and seventeen bronchoscopies and repeated infection, that was breathing room air again but doing so with the reserve capacity of someone decades older and considerably more compromised. A rhinovirus — a common cold — that would have meant two days of inconvenience for a healthy person could have meant a return to the hospital for Dave. Could have meant pneumonia. Could have meant something we did not want to contemplate.

Elderberry and echinacea together became the immune foundation of our household. Not just for Dave — for all of us. Because a cold that the girls brought home from school and shrugged off in three days was a cold that could reach Dave. We were all, in a sense, protecting him by protecting ourselves.

That is still true today. We all use it. At the first sign. Every time.

What the Research Actually Says

Elderberry is one of the most extensively researched medicinal plants in the modern botanical literature, which puts it in rare company. Most herbs are supported primarily by traditional use and emerging mechanistic research. Elderberry has randomized controlled trials — the gold standard of clinical evidence — and the results are consistent enough to have attracted attention from mainstream medical researchers who started out skeptical.

The berries of Sambucus nigra contain a remarkable concentration of anthocyanins — the deep purple pigments that give the fruit its color and that have documented antioxidant, anti-inflammatory, and antiviral properties. They also contain flavonoids, including quercetin and rutin, with independent antiviral and immune-modulating activity, along with vitamins A and C, zinc, and a range of phenolic compounds that collectively make elderberry one of the most nutritionally dense medicinal fruits available.

A 2016 randomized, double-blind, placebo-controlled study published in Nutrients found that elderberry supplementation substantially reduced the duration and severity of colds in air travelers — a population under significant immune stress. Those taking elderberry experienced colds that were on average two days shorter and significantly less severe than those taking placebo.

The mechanism behind these effects is increasingly well understood. Elderberry compounds appear to work in two complementary ways: they directly inhibit the ability of certain viruses to penetrate and replicate within host cells, and they modulate the immune response — stimulating cytokine production to mount a faster defense while simultaneously regulating the inflammatory response to prevent it from overshooting. This dual action is what makes elderberry particularly intelligent as an immune herb. It does not simply rev the immune system up indiscriminately. It helps the immune system do its job more efficiently and more precisely.

This distinction — between stimulating the immune system and modulating it — matters enormously for anyone whose immune system has been through what Dave's had. A depleted immune system does not need to be driven harder. It needs to be supported in working smarter. Elderberry, in our experience and in the research literature, does exactly that.

A Note on the Cytokine Storm Question

If you have read anything about elderberry in the last several years, you may have encountered concern about its potential to trigger or worsen a cytokine storm — the dangerous overactivation of the immune response associated with severe cases of influenza and, more recently, with COVID-19. This concern circulated widely during the pandemic and caused many people to stop using elderberry out of caution.

I want to address this directly, because the concern deserves a careful answer rather than dismissal or blind reassurance.

The cytokine storm hypothesis around elderberry was based primarily on its known ability to stimulate cytokine production — the reasoning being that if cytokines cause the storm, and elderberry increases cytokines, elderberry might worsen the storm. This is a logical chain that does not hold up under closer examination. The cytokines elderberry stimulates are primarily those involved in the early innate immune response — the rapid first-line defense that, when functioning well, actually prevents the kind of uncontrolled viral replication that leads to cytokine storm in the first place. The research on elderberry's immunomodulatory effects suggests it helps regulate the immune response rather than simply amplifying it without limit.

As always, anyone managing a serious immune condition, taking immunosuppressive medications, or dealing with a severe acute illness should consult with a qualified healthcare practitioner before using any herbal preparation, including elderberry. That is not a caveat I add out of legal habit. It is something I genuinely mean, as someone who has navigated exactly that territory.

On Tea Bags and Why They Do Not Belong Here

Before I give you the recipes for elderberry, I want to say something that applies to every herb in this reference but that I want to say here, plainly, because elderberry is so widely available in pre-packaged commercial form that the temptation to cut corners is real.

I do not buy any herbs that are pre-made in a tea bag. I only buy my herbs from the herb farm. That is not a preference. That is a standard. And it is one I want every reader of this book to understand and adopt.

A commercial tea bag is not medicine. It is often the lowest grade of the herb — the dust and broken fragments left after the quality material has been sorted out — stored in a warehouse for an indeterminate period, packaged in a bag that may be sealed with epichlorohydrin, a compound classified as a possible carcinogen, or made from plastic-based materials that release microplastics into hot water. The very act of steeping — which you do specifically to extract compounds from the plant into the water — also extracts whatever the bag is made of.

You rebuilt every shelf in your house. Do not put a commercial tea bag in the hot water you are drinking for your health.

Whole dried elderberries from a trusted farm. A proper tincture made by people who know this plant. That is what belongs in this protocol. The difference in quality, potency, and safety is not subtle.

At the first sign of illness — the scratchy throat, the sudden fatigue — Elderberry tincture was the first thing off the counter. Combined always with Echinacea. Sourced from the farm. Not a commercial preparation. Whole plant material, properly extracted, recently made.

A note on timing that I cannot emphasize enough: the window in which elderberry and echinacea are most effective is the first few hours of immune challenge — before the virus has replicated to the point where the immune system is playing catch-up. This is why the tincture lives on the counter, not in a cabinet. This is why we act immediately rather than waiting to see how bad it gets.

In a household with a man whose lungs spent five months on a ventilator, waiting to see how bad a cold gets was never an option. That urgency shaped a protocol that has served our whole family well for years. The first sign is the right time. Not the second sign. Not when you are sure. The first whisper of something coming is exactly when these herbs are most useful.

Keep them where you can reach them without thinking. That is the whole instruction.

Garlic

Allium sativum | *The Medicine That Feeds You*

There is an argument to be made that garlic is the most medicinal food in the average kitchen — not herb cabinet, not supplement shelf, kitchen. It is in the vegetable drawer. It costs almost nothing. It has been used as medicine by virtually every culture on earth that had access to it. And the gap between what most people understand garlic to be — a flavoring, a culinary staple, something that makes food taste better — and what it actually does inside the body is one of the largest gaps in popular nutritional understanding.

In our household garlic works three ways simultaneously, and I want to name all three before I explain any of them: as an antimicrobial and antiviral for immune support, as a cardiovascular herb for blood pressure and circulation, and as part of the antiparasitic protocol that is covered in full in Chapter Four of this book. Three distinct applications, one bulb, one kitchen, one house that had decided food was medicine and meant it literally.

We use it as a tincture from the farm for concentrated therapeutic support, and we cook with it in everything savory — which in a house where Celtic sea salt and black pepper go into every cooked dish means garlic is present at almost every meal. That daily culinary exposure is not incidental. It is a sustained, low-dose protocol that runs underneath and alongside the concentrated tincture use, and the two together provide a depth of coverage that neither provides alone.

> *Garlic has been found in Egyptian tombs dating to 3000 BCE, prescribed in the Ebers Papyrus for twenty-two separate conditions. It appears in the oldest surviving medical texts of India, China, Greece, and Rome. When every independent healing tradition on earth reaches for the same food across five thousand years, the appropriate response is to pay attention.*

Allicin — The Compound That Does the Work

Fresh garlic does not contain allicin. It contains alliin, a sulfur compound that is converted to allicin by the enzyme alliinase when the cell walls of the garlic are disrupted — by crushing, chopping, chewing, or pressing. This conversion is the most practically important fact about using garlic medicinally, because it means that whole uncrushed garlic — swallowed as a supplement or added whole to cooking — does not produce the same therapeutic compounds as garlic that has been properly prepared.

Crush it. Chop it. Let it sit for ten minutes after crushing before cooking with it — the alliinase reaction continues during that window and produces more allicin than immediate heat exposure would allow. That ten-minute rest is a small act with a meaningful biochemical consequence.

Allicin is one of the most broadly antimicrobial natural compounds identified in the research literature. Studies have documented activity against a wide spectrum of bacteria, including antibiotic-resistant strains like MRSA, against fungi including Candida species, against viruses including influenza, and against parasites including Giardia and several species of intestinal helminths. The mechanism involves allicin's ability to inhibit sulfhydryl-containing enzymes essential to pathogen metabolism — a mechanism that pathogens have not developed significant resistance to, in contrast to many pharmaceutical antibiotics.

For Dave, coming home from six months of broad-spectrum antibiotic use that had disrupted his microbiome and potentially created conditions hospitable to opportunistic organisms, garlic's broad antimicrobial range was specifically relevant. Not as a replacement for medical treatment of any identified infection, but as a daily food-level exposure to compounds that create an inhospitable environment for the opportunistic organisms that proliferate in a disrupted microbiome.

Garlic and the Cardiovascular System

The cardiovascular research on garlic is among the most extensive in the herbal medicine literature, spanning decades and hundreds of clinical studies. The consistent findings across this body of research document garlic's ability to modestly but meaningfully reduce blood pressure, reduce LDL cholesterol oxidation, inhibit platelet aggregation — the clumping that contributes to clot formation — and reduce arterial stiffness and inflammation in the endothelial lining of blood vessels.

For Dave, whose cardiovascular system had been through a cardiac event during his MICU stay and whose heart was recovering alongside everything else, gentle, sustained cardiovascular support was not a luxury. The endothelial lining of blood vessels — the thin cellular layer that regulates vascular tone, prevents clotting, and governs the inflammatory response in vessel walls — is among the tissues most affected by prolonged critical illness and the inflammatory cascade it generates. Garlic's documented anti-inflammatory and endothelial-protective effects made it a specific and logical choice for daily long-term cardiovascular support.

This is also where the cooking application earns its place medicinally rather than just culinarily. The daily inclusion of properly prepared garlic — crushed, rested, then cooked — in bone broth, in soups, in roasted vegetables, in everything savory provides a consistent low-dose cardiovascular exposure that accumulates over weeks and months into something meaningful. It is not the acute dose of the tincture. It is the steady, daily presence of a food that the cardiovascular system benefits from encountering regularly.

Garlic and the Antiparasitic Protocol

The third application of garlic in our household is the one least often discussed in mainstream herbal literature and the one most central to the philosophy of root-cause thinking that runs through this entire book: its role in the antiparasitic protocol.

Garlic's antiparasitic properties have been documented in both traditional use across multiple cultures and in modern research. Allicin and its derivatives have demonstrated activity against Giardia lamblia, Trypanosoma species, and several intestinal helminths in laboratory and clinical research. The mechanism involves the same sulfhydryl enzyme inhibition that makes garlic antimicrobial — disrupting the metabolic processes of parasitic organisms in ways that do not similarly affect human cells.

In the context of this book, garlic is one component of a broader antiparasitic and gut-restoration protocol that is discussed in full in Chapter Four — the root cause chapter that examines why the body becomes hospitable to parasitic organisms in the first place and what a comprehensive approach to addressing that looks like. Garlic alone is not the protocol. It is one thread in it, running consistently through the daily food and the concentrated tincture use, creating the kind of sustained unfavorable environment for opportunistic organisms that a single aggressive treatment cannot replicate.

The daily presence of garlic in the food is, in this sense, both medicine and prevention simultaneously. The kitchen as the first line of defense. Which is, at its core, what this entire book is about.

I want to be specific here, because the protocol was not random. Dave had survived sepsis and candida in the bloodstream while on ECMO — weeks of systemic infection while his body was being kept alive by a machine. The gut that comes home after that is not simply depleted. It has been stripped. Burdock Root for the lymphatic and gut rebuilding. Garlic for its antifungal and antimicrobial properties — the pharmaceutical protocol had addressed the infection chemically, but left no plan to restore what it had taken. These were not casual choices. They were the answer to a specific history.

We used Garlic two ways simultaneously — as a tincture from the farm for concentrated therapeutic support, and in the kitchen every day. Crushed, rested for ten minutes to activate the allicin, then cooked into bone broth, soups, and everything savory.

Medicine that feeds you. Food that heals you. The distinction between the two, in a kitchen that has decided what it is for, disappears entirely.

Body Systems: Immune | Cardiovascular | Antimicrobial | Digestive

Ailments: Immune Support, Viral and Bacterial Infection, Blood Pressure, Cardiovascular Recovery, Antiparasitic Protocol, Post-Antibiotic Microbiome Restoration

Hawthorn

Crataegus monogyna, C. laevigata | *The Heart's Herb*

Dave had a cardiac event during his time in the MICU.

I am going to say that plainly, without softening it, because it deserves to be said plainly. He had already survived ECMO. He had survived a tracheostomy and seventeen bronchoscopies and dialysis and five months on a ventilator. And somewhere in the middle of all of that, his heart — the muscle that had been working under extraordinary metabolic stress, in a body depleted of the minerals and oxygen and rest that cardiac tissue depends on — had its own crisis.

He survived that too. But a heart that has been through what his heart went through does not simply return to baseline when the acute event is over. It carries the history of what happened to it. It needs specific, sustained, intelligent support while it recovers — support that addresses the heart muscle itself, the blood pressure regulation that prolonged illness and prolonged medication use leave dysregulated, the circulatory system that delivers oxygen and nutrients to every cell in the body, and the inflammation in the vascular endothelium that critical illness generates and that persists long after discharge.

Hawthorn is the herb for all of that. And it is, in my view, the most important cardiovascular herb in the Western botanical tradition — the one with the deepest research base, the most specific cardiac affinity, and the most consistent record of meaningful benefit in exactly the conditions Dave's heart was navigating.

> *There is a concept in traditional herbalism called organ affinity — the idea that certain herbs have a specific relationship with certain organs, addressing them more directly and more intelligently than their general biochemical profile would suggest. Hawthorn's affinity for the heart is one of the most thoroughly documented examples of this concept in the entire botanical world.*

What Hawthorn Does for the Heart

Hawthorn — the berries, flowers, and leaves of Crataegus species — contains one of the most impressive concentrations of cardiovascular-active compounds in the plant world. Oligomeric proanthocyanidins, vitexin, quercetin, hyperoside, and a range of flavonoids work through multiple simultaneous mechanisms to support cardiac function in ways that have been the subject of serious clinical investigation for decades.

The primary mechanisms, as the research currently understands them, include: dilation of the coronary arteries, increasing blood flow to the heart muscle itself; improvement of the heart's contractile efficiency, allowing it to do more work with less oxygen consumption; reduction of peripheral vascular resistance, which reduces the workload on the heart; anti-inflammatory and antioxidant effects in the endothelial lining of blood vessels; and mild antihypertensive effects through multiple pathways.

The Heart After Critical Illness

The cardiac complications of prolonged critical illness are well documented and consistently underappreciated in the post-discharge recovery conversation. The heart that has been working under the metabolic stress of critical illness — through hypoxia, through systemic inflammation, through the cardiovascular demands of ECMO and vasopressor support and the fluid shifts of critical illness — is not the same heart that was admitted to the ICU.

Myocardial stunning — transient impairment of cardiac contractile function following periods of reduced oxygen supply — is common in critical illness even in patients without pre-existing cardiac disease. Inflammatory damage to the cardiac endothelium accumulates during prolonged systemic inflammation.

Micronutrient depletion — of magnesium, potassium, CoQ10, and the B vitamins essential to cardiac metabolism — occurs during critical illness faster than it can be replaced through standard ICU nutrition.

The heart that came home in September 2021 needed time, and it needed specific support. Not aggressive intervention — Dave was working with his medical team on the pharmaceutical aspects of his cardiovascular recovery. What the pharmaceutical protocol does not provide is the gentle, sustained, trophorestorative support for the cardiac tissue itself that herbal medicine has been offering for centuries and that the clinical research increasingly validates.

Hawthorn is a trophorestorative herb for the heart — meaning it does not simply manage symptoms or force a physiological response, but over time restores tone, function, and resilience to cardiac tissue that has been depleted or damaged. That distinction matters. Dave's heart did not need to be driven harder. It needed to be nourished back to strength.

Blood Pressure, Circulation, and the Long Recovery

Blood pressure dysregulation is one of the most common and most persistent cardiovascular sequelae of prolonged critical illness. The medications used in the ICU to maintain hemodynamic stability —

vasopressors, sedatives, corticosteroids — each affect vascular tone in ways that can leave blood pressure regulation impaired for months after discharge. The autonomic nervous system, which governs blood pressure moment-to-moment, is itself affected by the prolonged stress of critical illness and the neurological consequences of PICS.

Hawthorn's gentle antihypertensive effects, working through vasodilation and endothelial support rather than through central nervous system suppression, made it specifically appropriate for this context. Not replacing the pharmaceutical management that Dave's cardiologist was overseeing. Complementing it — working through different mechanisms to support the vascular system's own capacity to regulate itself, which is ultimately what recovery means.

For peripheral circulation — the blood flow to the extremities that critical illness, prolonged immobility, and cardiac compromise all reduce — Hawthorn's vasodilatory properties support exactly the kind of improved peripheral circulation that aids tissue healing, reduces the cold extremities that many post-ICU patients experience, and supports the gradual return of stamina and physical capacity that defines the recovery arc.

We use Hawthorn as a tincture from the farm, taken daily as an ongoing cardiovascular support. It is one of the herbs in this reference that I think of as permanent — not something to take for a period and then stop, but something that belongs in the long-term protocol for anyone whose heart has been through significant stress and is engaged in the slow, unannounced work of finding its way back to full strength.

Hawthorn was Dave's daily cardiac tonic — taken consistently for months as a tincture from the farm. The cardiovascular stress of his MICU stay required something slow, steady, and cumulative. Hawthorn is exactly that.

The heart that survived deserves a protocol worthy of what it endured. Hawthorn is part of that protocol. It has been since he came home. It will be for as long as we have reason to be grateful, which is to say for the rest of our lives.

Body Systems: Cardiovascular | Circulatory | Blood Pressure | Vascular

Ailments: Post-Cardiac Event Recovery, Blood Pressure Regulation, Heart Failure Support, Circulatory Insufficiency, Peripheral Circulation, Post-ICU Cardiovascular Recovery, Endothelial Health

Ginger

There are herbs in this reference that required research to find and effort to source. Ginger is not one of them. It is in every grocery store on earth, in every cuisine on every continent, and has been used medicinally for more than five thousand years across cultures that had no contact with each other and independently reached the same conclusions about what this root could do.

That kind of convergence is not coincidence. It is evidence.

Ginger is one of the most pharmacologically active foods available to the human kitchen — a root whose compounds address nausea, inflammation, circulation, digestion, and immune defense simultaneously, in forms that range from a thin raw slice chewed slowly to a concentrated tincture from a trusted farm. It is the herb we reach for when someone feels nauseous, when digestion is sluggish, when circulation needs warming, when a cold is threatening, and when heartburn arrives — that last use always alongside Marshmallow Root, whose profile follows this one for exactly that reason.

We use it all of us, depending on what the situation calls for. Tincture from the farm for concentrated support. Fresh root because sometimes the most direct route is the best one — a thin slice of raw ginger, chewed slowly, is one of the fastest-acting nausea remedies that exists. And ginger appears regularly in our cooking because a kitchen that has already decided food is medicine finds natural allies in ingredients that are both delicious and bioactive.

> *Ginger root, eaten raw, contains gingerol in its most potent form — the compound responsible for the majority of its medicinal activity, before heat or drying converts it to other forms. When nausea arrives and you need something that works quickly, a thin slice of fresh ginger chewed slowly is not a folk remedy. It is pharmacology you can grow in a pot on the windowsill.*

What Ginger Actually Does

The primary active compounds in fresh ginger are gingerols — phenolic compounds concentrated in the fresh root that are responsible for its characteristic sharp heat and the majority of its therapeutic activity. When ginger is dried, gingerols convert to shogaols, which are more pungent and have their own distinct medicinal properties, particularly for nausea and anti-inflammatory action. When cooked, a portion converts to paradols and zingerone. Each form of ginger is slightly different medicinally, which is why using it in multiple forms — fresh, tincture, dried in cooking — captures the broadest range of its activity.

The anti-nausea mechanism is one of the most thoroughly documented in botanical medicine. Ginger compounds act on the gastrointestinal tract directly, reducing the hypersensitivity of gastric smooth muscle and accelerating gastric emptying — which addresses one of the primary causes of both nausea and the reflux that produces heartburn. They also act centrally, on the serotonin receptors in the gut and brain that mediate nausea signals, in ways that overlap with pharmaceutical anti-nausea medications but without their sedative and neurological side effects.

The research on Ginger and nausea is among the most consistent in botanical medicine — multiple studies, multiple conditions, comparable results to the standard pharmaceutical approach and without the side effects. I did not need a meta-analysis to tell me this. I needed it to tell Dave's doctors.

The anti-inflammatory mechanism overlaps with turmeric's — ginger also inhibits NF-κB and prostaglandin synthesis — which is why the two herbs are often used together and why both are in the cooking in this house. Together they address inflammation from complementary angles, and the combination has been used in Ayurvedic medicine for centuries under exactly that rationale.

Ginger and Heartburn — The Motility Connection

Heartburn is one of the most commonly misunderstood digestive conditions in conventional medicine, and ginger's role in addressing it is one of the clearest illustrations of why treating the cause produces better results than suppressing the symptom.

The standard pharmaceutical approach to heartburn — antacids, H2 blockers, proton pump inhibitors — reduces stomach acid production. This addresses the burning sensation but creates a downstream problem: stomach acid is not the enemy. It is essential. Adequate stomach acid is required for protein digestion, for mineral absorption, for killing pathogens that enter through the mouth, and for signaling the lower esophageal sphincter to close properly. Reduce stomach acid significantly or chronically and you impair all of those functions simultaneously.

In many cases of heartburn and reflux, the underlying issue is not too much stomach acid but delayed gastric emptying — food sitting in the stomach longer than it should, creating pressure that pushes whatever acid is present upward into the esophagus. Ginger addresses this directly by improving gastric motility — the movement of food through the digestive system — through its effect on gastric smooth muscle.

Move the food through faster, reduce the pressure, and the acid stays where it belongs.

We use ginger tincture for Dave's heartburn alongside Marshmallow Root — always the two together. Ginger to improve the motility that is the root cause. Marshmallow Root to soothe the esophageal tissue that has been irritated. One addresses the mechanism, the other supports the healing of the tissue that has been affected. That combination is covered in full in the Marshmallow Root profile that follows this one.

For anyone who has been on proton pump inhibitors long-term and is concerned about what that means for their digestion, mineral absorption, and gut microbiome — the questions in this section are worth bringing to a qualified integrative practitioner. The relationship between stomach acid, gut health, and long-term pharmaceutical acid suppression is a conversation this book cannot fully contain, but it is one worth having.

Ginger After Prolonged Hospitalization

There is a specific application of ginger's motility-improving properties that is rarely discussed in the context of post-ICU recovery but that was directly relevant to Dave's situation: the gut that has been on tube feeding for months.

Prolonged enteral nutrition — tube feeding — bypasses the normal digestive process in ways that leave the gut's own motility mechanisms underused and often significantly impaired. The migrating motor complex — the wave-like muscular contractions that move food and waste through the digestive tract — atrophies without regular use. The result, in many post-ICU patients, is a digestive system that does not move food through efficiently, producing bloating, discomfort, constipation, and the kind of general digestive sluggishness that Dave experienced in the early weeks at home.

A thin slice of fresh ginger before meals. A cup of ginger tea made from real root. A few drops of tincture in water. In our experience these simple, immediate interventions made a noticeable difference in digestive comfort during the months when Dave's gut was relearning how to work.

Ginger worked alongside Marshmallow Root for Dave's digestive recovery — the gut that had spent months on tube feeding and needed to relearn its own function. We used it as a tincture from the farm, often combined with Marshmallow Root.

Keep fresh ginger root in the refrigerator at all times — it keeps for several weeks and costs almost nothing.

Suggested Use:

Ginger has been in the human medicine chest longer than almost any herb in this reference. Five thousand years of the same reach, across cultures that never spoke to each other, for the same root. The stomach that will not settle. The hands that will not warm. The cold coming on. The circulation that needs moving.

It works in a kitchen drawer and it works in a tincture bottle and it works as a thin raw slice held in the mouth while nausea subsides. It is not glamorous. It does not have ten thousand published studies behind it the way Turmeric does. What it has is something more durable than research: it has the accumulated agreement of every healing tradition that ever touched it, saying quietly and consistently, across five millennia: this one works.

Keep fresh ginger in your refrigerator. Always. The rest is details.

Body Systems: Digestive | Circulatory | Immune | Anti-inflammatory

Ailments: Nausea, Heartburn, Digestive Sluggishness, Cold Hands and Feet, Post-Hospital Gut Recovery, Cold and Flu, Inflammation, Poor Circulation

Marshmallow Root

Althaea officinalis | *The Great Soother*

There is a category of herbs called demulcents — from the Latin demulcere, to stroke gently — and Marshmallow Root is the most complete example of this category in the Western botanical tradition. A demulcent herb coats, soothes, and protects irritated or inflamed mucous membranes, creating a physical barrier that allows damaged tissue to rest and heal while protecting it from further irritation.

It sounds simple. The clinical implications are not.

Every surface in the body lined with mucous membrane — the mouth, the throat, the esophagus, the stomach, the intestines, the urinary tract, the respiratory passages — is a potential site where Marshmallow Root's demulcent action is relevant. And when you consider what Dave's body had been through — intubation for five months, a tracheostomy, seventeen bronchoscopies, tube feeding, months of pharmaceutical exposure, and the esophageal and gastric tissue that all of that leaves behind — the question is not whether Marshmallow Root belongs in this protocol. The question is why it took as long as it did to add it.

We use it specifically for heartburn — always alongside Ginger, always as a pair. And that pairing is

"

the most important thing to understand about Marshmallow Root's place in this reference: it does not address causes. It soothes consequences. Used alone for heartburn it provides relief but does not resolve the underlying motility issue that is generating the acid reflux. Used with Ginger, which does address the motility, it becomes part of a complete response — one herb moving the food through properly, the other soothing the tissue that the acid has irritated in the meantime.

> *That is the logic of combining herbs: not redundancy but complementarity. Each one doing something the other cannot. The whole greater than the sum of its parts. This is how traditional medicine has always worked, and it is how this protocol works.*

The Mucilage and What It Does

The active constituent responsible for Marshmallow Root's demulcent action is mucilage — a complex of polysaccharides that, when hydrated, forms a thick, gel-like substance that coats mucous membranes on contact. This is not metaphorical coating. It is physical. The mucilage adheres to the surface of irritated tissue, creating a protective layer that reduces friction, blocks the contact of acidic or irritating substances with the underlying cells, and allows the tissue's own repair mechanisms to work without constant reinjury.

The anti-inflammatory compounds in Marshmallow Root — including flavonoids and phenolic acids — work alongside the physical mucilage to reduce the inflammatory response in the underlying tissue, accelerating healing rather than simply masking discomfort. Research has documented Marshmallow Root's efficacy for pharyngitis — throat inflammation — with a study published in Complementary Medicine Research finding significant reduction in throat irritation and pain in participants using a Marshmallow Root syrup compared to placebo.

For the esophagus specifically — the tissue most directly affected by acid reflux — Marshmallow Root's mucilage coats the esophageal lining in a way that provides immediate relief from the burning sensation while the underlying tissue heals. This is why it works so well in combination with Ginger reduces the acid exposure by improving motility, Marshmallow Root protects and heals the tissue that has already been exposed.

Beyond the esophagus and stomach, Marshmallow Root has a long and well-documented history of use for the urinary tract — soothing the lining of the bladder and urethra in urinary tract infections, reducing the burning and urgency that make UTIs so miserable, and creating an environment less hospitable to the bacterial adhesion that sustains infection. It has been used for respiratory mucous membranes — the bronchial lining that Mullein addresses structurally, Marshmallow Root soothes when inflamed or irritated. And it has been used for intestinal inflammation, including in conditions like irritable bowel syndrome and leaky gut, where the integrity of the intestinal lining is compromised.

For a body that had been intubated for five months, that had a tracheostomy, that had seventeen bronchoscopies passing instruments through airways, that had tube feeding running through the esophagus — the mucous membranes of the entire respiratory and digestive tract had been through a level of physical trauma that most bodies never experience. Marshmallow Root, used consistently, addresses the healing of that tissue at a level that no pharmaceutical in the discharge paperwork had even acknowledged as a need.

A Note on Preparation — Cold Infusion

Marshmallow Root requires a specific preparation note that distinguishes it from almost every other herb in this reference: its mucilage is best extracted in cold water, not hot.

Heat degrades a portion of the mucilaginous polysaccharides that are responsible for the demulcent action. A cold infusion — root steeped in room temperature or cold water for several hours or overnight — extracts the mucilage more completely and produces a more viscous, more soothing preparation than a hot tea. The result looks different from most herb teas: thick, slightly viscous, almost silky in texture. That thickness is the medicine. It is what coats the tissue.

The tincture we use from the farm handles this through the extraction process. For anyone making their own preparation at home, the cold infusion method is the approach that delivers the full demulcent action.

Every surface the hospital had traumatized — the throat, the esophagus, the respiratory passages — was a site where Marshmallow Root had something to offer. We used a tincture from the farm, sometimes combined with Ginger for digestive support.

Sometimes the most sophisticated thing medicine can do is get out of the way and let tissue heal. Marshmallow Root holds the space for that to happen.

Body Systems: Digestive | Respiratory | Urinary | Mucosal Lining

Ailments: Heartburn, Acid Reflux, Esophageal Irritation, Urinary Tract Infection, Gut Lining Support, Post-Intubation Recovery, Throat Inflammation, IBS

Milk Thistle

Ask most people to name a liver herb, and if they know one at all, it is this one. Milk Thistle has become something of a celebrity in the world of natural medicine — and unlike many celebrities, it has earned its reputation.

The plant itself is striking: a tall, spiny thistle with leaves marbled in silver-white, as though someone traced their fingers through them in cream. It is native to the Mediterranean but now grows on nearly every continent, thriving on roadsides and disturbed ground with the cheerful persistence of something that knows it belongs wherever healing is needed.

The active compound responsible for most of Milk Thistle's documented effects is a flavonoid complex called silymarin, found primarily in the seeds. Silymarin is, in essence, a hepatoprotective — a liver protector. It works through several mechanisms simultaneously: it stabilizes cell membranes in the liver, reducing the uptake of toxins; it stimulates the production of new liver cells to replace damaged ones; and it acts as a powerful antioxidant, neutralizing the free radicals that inflammatory processes generate.

In Herbal Medicine: Expanded Commission E Monographs, pharmacognosist Mark Blumenthal notes that Milk Thistle seed extract has been the subject of more than 30 controlled clinical trials, making it one of the most rigorously studied herbs in Western botanical medicine. The German Commission E — a scientific advisory body considered among the world's most thorough evaluators of herbal medicines — approved Milk Thistle for use in toxic liver damage, chronic inflammatory liver disease, and cirrhosis.

For Dave, the liver connection was not incidental. One of the lesser-discussed realities of prolonged pharmaceutical treatment — the kind that comes with extended hospital stays, with antibiotics layered on immunosuppressants layered on pain management — is the cumulative burden placed on the liver. The organ responsible for processing every substance that enters the body was, after months of intensive medical care, working harder than it was designed to sustain. Milk Thistle became one of the first herbs I reached for, and one of the last I set down.

There is also an emerging body of research connecting liver health to the broader terrain of the body — including the gut microbiome, inflammatory pathways, and immune regulation. Dr. Aviva Romm, whose book Botanical Medicine for Women's Health bridges clinical medicine and traditional herbalism with rare sophistication, describes the liver as a central clearinghouse for the body's toxic load. When it is overburdened, everything downstream suffers.

This raises a question worth sitting with: how often are symptoms we treat in isolation — fatigue, brain fog, skin issues, hormonal imbalance — downstream consequences of a liver that simply cannot keep up? Modern medicine excels at addressing the symptom. Milk Thistle asks us to consider the source.

As always, speak with your healthcare provider before introducing any new herb, particularly if you are managing a diagnosed liver condition or taking pharmaceuticals metabolized by the liver. Silymarin can affect the cytochrome P450 enzyme system, which processes many common medications.

I used Milk Thistle as a tincture throughout Dave's recovery — sourced from the farm, taken daily. After six months of antibiotics, antivirals, and sedatives, his liver needed sustained, gentle support. This was not optional. It was the foundation.

Body Systems: Liver & Gallbladder | Digestive | Immune | Skin

Ailments: Post-Pharmaceutical Liver Recovery, Toxic Liver Damage, Chronic Liver Disease, Pharmaceutical Burden, Immune Support, Skin Conditions

Lemon Balm

Melissa officinalis | *The Gentle Daily Presence*

There is a category of anxiety that does not announce itself dramatically. It does not arrive as panic. It does not produce obvious symptoms that would lead a doctor to write a prescription or a friend to notice something is wrong. It simply lives in the background of everything — a low hum of tension that is always present, that makes the stomach tight and the thoughts circular and the sleep light and the days heavier than they ought to be.

That is the anxiety that Lemon Balm is made for.

During the months of Dave's recovery at home — the oxygen concentrator humming in the corner, the pulse oximeter on the nightstand, my nervous system permanently tuned to the frequency of his breathing — my anxiety lived in all of those places at once. It was in my mind during the day, looping through the same questions on the same track. It was in my gut, which had been chronically tense for so long that I had stopped noticing it as a symptom and started accepting it as just how I felt. It was in my sleep, which was light and fragmented and populated with thoughts that would not quiet even when exhaustion finally pulled me under.

And it was in the daytime, in the hours when Dave was resting and the house was quiet and there was no immediate task to focus on — those hours were some of the hardest. The body that had been running on adrenaline and purpose for six months did not know what to do with stillness. Stillness felt like danger. Stillness felt like the moment before bad news.

And for Dave, simultaneously, it was addressing something completely different through exactly the same mechanism: the sluggish, bloated digestion of a gut that had spent months on tube feeding and was still learning, slowly, how to work again. The anxious gut and the recovering gut — different presentations, same herb, same underlying truth about how the nervous system and the digestive system are not separate things at all.

The Gut-Brain Connection — Why One Herb Does Both

The enteric nervous system — the network of neurons embedded in the gastrointestinal tract — contains more nerve cells than the spinal cord. It communicates bidirectionally with the brain through the vagus nerve in a relationship so intimate and so constant that researchers have begun calling the gut the second brain. This is not a metaphor. It is anatomy.

When the central nervous system is chronically activated — under sustained stress, in prolonged vigilance, in the aftermath of trauma — the enteric nervous system responds in kind. Motility slows or becomes erratic. Digestion becomes inefficient. Bloating, sluggishness, discomfort, and the general sense that the gut is not working the way it should — these are the digestive system expressing what the nervous system is experiencing. The gut is not malfunctioning independently. It is accurately reflecting the state of the nervous system it is connected to.

Lemon Balm addresses both ends of this connection simultaneously. Its anxiolytic compounds — rosmarinic acid, flavonoids including luteolin and apigenin, and volatile oils including citral and citronellol — act on the central nervous system to reduce anxiety and promote calm. Its antispasmodic properties act directly on the smooth muscle of the gastrointestinal tract, relaxing the tension that slows motility and causes bloating. You are not taking two herbs for two problems. You are taking one herb that addresses one interconnected system at both ends.

Lemon Balm has been tested in clinical trials for anxiety, depression, and insomnia — and it holds up. Not in the dramatic way pharmaceutical interventions hold up, with fast sedation and next-day fog. In the way that matters for daily life — consistently, gently, without cost to the body that takes it.

For digestive function specifically, Lemon Balm has been studied alongside Peppermint for functional dyspepsia — the bloating, the cramping, the sluggish digestion that does not respond to ordinary remedies. The combination works. The gut, it turns out, listens to the nervous system.

The research confirms what the body already knows: calm the nervous system and the gut follows. Relax the gut and the nervous system follows. Lemon Balm works in both directions at once, which is precisely why it served two people in this household for two completely different presentations of the same underlying truth.

The Herb of Lightness

Lemon Balm — Melissa officinalis, its genus name derived from the Greek word for honey bee, because bees are irresistibly drawn to its flowers — is a member of the mint family, native to the Mediterranean and western Asia and naturalized across temperate regions worldwide. It has been cultivated in monastery gardens since at least the Middle Ages, where it was used for melancholy, for the nervous heart, for the digestion that would not settle, and for the kind of low-grade anxiety that prolonged difficulty produces in people who are doing their best to hold things together.

The eleventh-century Persian physician Avicenna — whose Canon of Medicine has appeared in this reference before — wrote that Lemon Balm "causes the mind and heart to become merry" and recommended it for palpitations, melancholy, and digestive disorders simultaneously. The sixteenth-century herbalist John Gerard called it "most comfortable for the heart." Paracelsus considered it one of the most valuable plants in his entire materia medica.

What all of these observers were describing, across centuries and traditions, is the same quality: Lemon Balm lifts. Not dramatically, not in the way that stimulants lift, not with the edge of something that will crash later. It lifts gently — the way a window opened in a room that has been closed too long lifts the air inside. You notice it as an absence of something heavy rather than the presence of something new. The circular thoughts slow. The gut unclenches. The day becomes slightly more possible than it was before.

That steadiness was what I needed during the months Dave was recovering at home. Not sedation — I could not afford sedation, I needed to be present and functional and capable of responding to anything that required responding to. I needed the background hum to quiet without the foreground going dark. Lemon Balm did that. Consistently, gently, without asking anything of me in return except that I take it.

Lemon Balm and the Post-Hospital Gut

Dave's digestive sluggishness in the months after coming home was not a mystery once I understood what his gut had been through. Six months of enteral nutrition — tube feeding that bypasses the normal digestive process entirely — followed by the reintroduction of real food to a system whose motility mechanisms had been largely dormant. Add the gut microbiome disruption from multiple courses of antibiotics. Add the effect of prolonged stress on intestinal motility through the gut-brain axis. Add the reduced physical activity of someone recovering from profound deconditioning.

The result is a digestive system that is sluggish, bloated, and uncomfortable in ways that do not respond to the things the average person might reach for — because those things address normal digestion, and what Dave had was not normal digestion. It was a system in the process of remembering how to work.

Lemon Balm, used consistently alongside Ginger — which we have already covered for its prokinetic properties — formed a gentle, sustained digestive support protocol that helped his gut find its rhythm again. Ginger to improve motility. Lemon Balm to relax the smooth muscle tension that was impeding it and to address the nervous system component that was contributing to the sluggishness. Together, in our experience, they made a meaningful difference in his comfort and in the efficiency of his digestion during those early months home.

For the Anxious Gut — A Note to Caregivers

I want to say something directly to anyone reading this who recognizes the anxiety-in-the-gut description from their own experience of caregiving or sustained stress.

The tight stomach that is always slightly clenched. The digestion that has been off for so long you have stopped thinking of it as a symptom. The nausea that arrives before difficult appointments or conversations. The bloating that appears during periods of high stress and resolves during rare periods of calm. This is your enteric nervous system expressing your central nervous system's state. It is not a separate digestive problem. It is an accurate and faithful reflection of what your nervous system is carrying.

Treating it as a digestive problem alone — with antacids, with fiber supplements, with dietary adjustments that help slightly but never fully resolve it — misses the root. The root is the nervous system. Address the nervous system and the gut follows. Not immediately, not overnight, but over weeks of consistent gentle support, the gut begins to reflect the calmer state you are trying to cultivate.

Lemon Balm is one of the kindest tools available for this. It does not demand anything difficult. It does not require a major lifestyle change or a course of treatment that takes months to complete. It is a tincture from a trusted farm, taken in water, daily. That is a manageable ask for someone who is already managing everything else.

Lemon Balm was the herb I reached for every day during Dave's recovery at home — for both of us. For him, it addressed the digestive sluggishness of a gut rebuilding after six months of tube feeding. For me, it was the daily presence that kept the nervous system from running too hot. Tincture from the farm, morning and afternoon.

That is not a small thing. For someone managing a recovering household, a nervous system in overdrive, two daughters watching their mother carefully, and a man on oxygen in the next room — slightly more possible was sometimes everything.

Melissa. The honey bee herb. Sweet, gentle, persistent. It does not sting. It just keeps showing up, day after day, making the day a little lighter than it would have been without it. That is enough. In the middle of something unsurvivable, that is more than enough.

Body Systems: Nervous System | Digestive | Gut-Brain Axis | Sleep

Ailments: Anxiety, Daily Stress, Caregiver Burnout, Digestive Sluggishness, Bloating, IBS, Insomnia from Anxious Thoughts, Post-Hospital Gut Recovery, Gut-Brain Dysregulation

Mullein

Verbascum thapsus | *The Lung's Oldest Ally*

If you have ever driven past a vacant lot or a disturbed roadside and noticed a tall, silver-green spike rising improbably from the gravel — sometimes five, six, seven feet into the air — you have seen Mullein. It is not a subtle plant. It does not hide. It grows where other things struggle, in compacted soil and rocky terrain and the margins of places, and it grows with the quiet confidence of something that has been doing this for a very long time.

Mullein has been used as a lung herb for more than two thousand years. The ancient Greeks documented it. Dioscorides, the first-century physician whose work De Materia Medica remained the foundational text of Western herbalism for fifteen centuries, wrote of its use for respiratory conditions. The Romans reportedly dipped the dried stalks in tallow and used them as torches — which is how Mullein acquired one of its many folk names: hag's taper. Native American peoples across dozens of nations used it independently for chest complaints, often smoking the dried leaves to open constricted airways. The Amish have used it. The Appalachian healers used it. Every tradition that had access to this plant, across cultures and centuries and continents, reached for it when someone couldn't breathe.

That kind of consensus across independent traditions is not something to dismiss lightly. It is, in the language of evidence, a signal.

The plant that arrived in North America with European colonists — considered a weed, naturalized so thoroughly it now grows in every U.S. state — carries in its soft, silvery leaves a remarkable concentration of compounds that explain what healers across history observed empirically. Saponins, which act as expectorants, loosening and thinning mucus so the lungs can clear it. Mucilage, which coats and soothes irritated mucous membranes throughout the respiratory tract. Flavonoids including verbascoside, which carry anti-inflammatory and antioxidant properties. And iridoids, which contribute to the plant's broader antimicrobial activity.

For Dave, coming home after five months on a ventilator with bilateral pneumonia and a formal diagnosis of chronic respiratory failure, the relevance was immediate and specific. His airways had been through extraordinary trauma — intubated, repeatedly bronchoscoped, subject to the kind of prolonged mechanical intervention that leaves tissue inflamed and the mucociliary clearance system — the lungs' own self-cleaning mechanism — significantly compromised.

Mullein addresses all of it. It soothes. It expectorates. It reduces inflammation. It supports the slow, effortful work of a respiratory system trying to remember how to function on its own.

In her foundational text Healing Wise, herbalist Susun Weed describes Mullein as "one of the best herbs for the lungs," noting its particular value in chronic respiratory conditions where the tissue is exhausted rather than acutely infected. That distinction matters. Acute infection is medicine's territory — and medicine handled Dave's acute phase with everything it had. But the long, slow rebuild of damaged tissue? That is where plants like Mullein have always lived.

A question worth sitting with: if the lungs are a bellows — designed to expand and contract, to move air and clear debris — what does months of mechanical ventilation do to a bellows that has not moved under its own power? And what does a plant that has been soothing inflamed airways for two millennia offer a bellows that is learning, slowly, painfully, to work again?

Mullein also carries a quieter gift that does not appear in pharmacological analyses: it is, visually and texturally, one of the most comforting plants in the botanical world. The leaves are thick and extraordinarily soft — softer than flannel, softer than most things — covered in fine silvery hairs that give the whole plant its characteristic pale glow. There is an old folk use of Mullein leaves as a chest poultice, laid directly on the skin over the lungs, and whether or not the compounds penetrate transdermally in meaningful quantities, the act of laying something that soft and warm over a chest that has been through what Dave's chest had been through is not nothing. The body knows when it is being tended.

Mullein was first — always first. A man coming home after five months on a ventilator with bilateral pneumonia needed his lungs supported above everything else. Daily tea from whole dried leaf, strained carefully through cheesecloth, taken warm every morning. Mullein tincture from the farm for additional support during acute episodes.

A note for the reader who is where I was: if someone you love has just come home from the hospital with compromised lungs — whether from COVID-19, pneumonia, COPD, or any other cause — Mullein tea is one of the gentlest, safest, most time-tested places to begin. It will not interfere with their medications. It will not overwhelm a body that is already overwhelmed. It will simply offer the lungs something that two thousand years of healers, working independently across every corner of the world, agreed they needed.

Start there. Start with the tea. Start with something warm and soft and ancient, and let the body do what bodies do when they are properly tended.

Body Systems: Respiratory | Ailments: Bronchitis, Chronic Cough, Post-Viral Lung Recovery, Asthma, Pleurisy

Nettle

Urtica dioica | *The Sting That Heals*

Most people's first encounter with Nettle is involuntary and unpleasant. The fine hollow hairs that cover the leaves and stems inject formic acid, histamine, and serotonin on contact, producing a sharp sting and a raised welt that can last for hours. It is the kind of plant that leaves an impression.

It also leaves an impression when you discover what it is capable of once properly prepared. Because the same plant that stings you in the garden — dried, tinctures, or cooked — is one of the most nutritionally dense, anti-inflammatory, allergy-relieving, kidney-supporting herbs in the entire botanical world. The sting and the medicine are not contradictions. They are the same plant showing you two different faces of the same fundamental truth: Nettle is potent. Respect it, and it will work for you in ways that will make you wonder why you ever reached for an antihistamine.

In our household, Nettle replaced antihistamines. For all of us. That is not a casual claim and I do not make it casually. It is what happened when we stopped suppressing the symptom and started addressing what was causing it.

Seasonal allergies — the sneezing, the itching, the streaming eyes, the fog of histamine response that descends every spring and lingers through summer — are an immune phenomenon. The body encounters a pollen or an environmental trigger and mounts an inflammatory response that releases histamine from mast cells, producing the familiar cascade of misery. Conventional antihistamines address this by blocking the H1 histamine receptor after the histamine has already been released — a downstream intervention that suppresses the symptom while doing nothing about the upstream inflammatory process that generated it.

Nettle works differently. Its active compounds — particularly quercetin, caffeic malic acid, and a range of flavonoids — inhibit the inflammatory enzymes and signaling pathways that produce the histamine response in the first place. It does not block the receptor after the fact. It reduces the conditions that trigger the response upstream. That is not a subtle distinction. It is the difference between treating a symptom and addressing its cause — which is, in essence, the philosophy of this entire book.

> *What that study does not capture, and what I want to say plainly: antihistamines carry costs that most people taking them daily through allergy season have never been told*

I am not a physician and I am not telling you to stop any medication without consulting your healthcare provider. What I am telling you is what I did for my family when I understood this — and what has worked, consistently, across multiple allergy seasons, for all of us.

Nettle tincture. From the farm. Started two to three weeks before allergy season begins, continued through the peak exposure period. In our experience — and in the research literature on its mechanism — the key is consistency and timing. Nettle works best as a preventive and ongoing support rather than as an acute rescue remedy. You are not suppressing a symptom when it arrives. You are reducing the inflammatory tendency that creates the symptom before it has a chance to fully develop.

The Nutritional Dimension

Seasonal allergies and kidney support are the two reasons we reach for Nettle most consistently — but they do not begin to capture what this plant actually contains. Nettle is, by almost any measure, one of the most nutritionally complete plants available to the human diet. It contains iron in concentrations that rival many animal sources, along with calcium, magnesium, potassium, phosphorus, and silica. It is rich in vitamins A, C, and K. It contains all nine essential amino acids — making it, unusually for a plant, a complete protein source.

For Dave, coming home with the nutritional depletion that follows six months of ICU nutrition — tube feeding, parenteral nutrition, and the metabolic demands of critical illness that consume micronutrients faster than they can be replaced — Nettle's mineral density was not incidental. A body rebuilding muscle, bone density, immune function, and cellular integrity needs raw materials. Nettle provides them in a form the body recognizes and absorbs readily, without the digestive burden of supplements manufactured in a laboratory.

Susun Weed, whose foundational work Healing Wise has shaped herbalist practice for decades, writes that a strong Nettle infusion — steeped for four to eight hours in a quart of boiling water — is one of the most nutrient-dense preparations available from any plant source, providing levels of calcium, magnesium, and iron that compare favorably with pharmaceutical supplementation. She calls it nourishing herbal infusion, and the distinction from a simple tea is important: the long steep extracts minerals that a ten-minute steep does not reach.

Kidney and Urinary Support

The second reason Nettle earned a permanent place in our protocol is its kidney affinity — and for Dave, this was not a general wellness consideration. It was specific and urgent.

Dave's kidneys were on dialysis during his MICU stay. The acute kidney injury that necessitated dialysis was a consequence of the systemic inflammatory response, the medications required to keep him alive, and the circulatory compromise that prolonged critical illness produces. Kidneys that have been through acute injury and dialysis do not simply reset when the crisis passes. They recover — in many cases remarkably — but they carry the history of what happened to them, and they benefit from ongoing, gentle, specific support.

For a body that had been on dialysis, that had processed months of pharmaceuticals through kidneys under stress, that needed sustained gentle support rather than another acute intervention — Nettle was a logical and well-supported choice. It remains part of the protocol.

There is a pattern I notice in the herbs that have stayed on our counter the longest — Nettle, Milk

Thistle, Burdock Root, Mullein. They are not dramatic herbs. They do not produce immediate, obvious effects that make you certain something is happening. They work slowly, quietly, over weeks and months, reducing burden and restoring function in systems that have been carrying too much. That kind of medicine requires patience and consistency. It also, in my observation, produces the most durable results.

A Note on Antihistamines and the Question Worth Asking

I want to return to the antihistamine question for a moment, because I think it represents something larger than allergy management.

Antihistamines are taken by tens of millions of people, daily, for months at a time, every allergy season, often for years or decades. They are considered so safe that they are available without a prescription. Most people who take them have never been told that first-generation antihistamines cross the blood-brain barrier and have anticholinergic activity. Most people who take them have never been told about the dementia research. Most people who take them have never been asked whether the symptom they are suppressing might be addressable at its source.

This is not a criticism of the people who take them. It is an observation about a medical culture that is extraordinarily good at suppressing symptoms and considerably less focused on asking why the symptoms are occurring and what it would take to address that upstream.

Nettle does not answer every allergy question. Allergies are complex, individual, and sometimes require medical management that goes beyond what any herb can provide. But for the seasonal, environmental, histamine-driven allergy response that affects so many families every spring — it is worth knowing that a plant exists that addresses the inflammatory mechanism rather than simply blocking the receptor. It is worth trying, under the guidance of a practitioner if you are managing other conditions, before accepting that a daily antihistamine for six months of the year is simply how it has to be.

In our experience, it does not have to be.

Nettle replaced antihistamines in our household — for all of us. Tincture from the farm, started two to three weeks before allergy season, continued through peak exposure. For Dave specifically it also addressed the nutritional depletion that follows six months of ICU nutrition.

It just requires knowing which end to hold.

Ailments: Seasonal Allergies, Allergic Rhinitis, Kidney Support, Post-Dialysis Recovery, Nutritional Depletion, Urinary Tract Health, Anemia, Inflammatory Conditions

157

Rose Petals

Rosa damascena, Rosa centifolia, Rosa canina | *The Heart's Medicine*

I want to begin this profile with something that herb books rarely say plainly: beauty is medicine.

Not metaphorically. Not as a soft addendum to the real, serious work of healing. Literally — as in, the experience of beauty has measurable physiological effects on the human body. It lowers cortisol. It activates the parasympathetic nervous system. It reduces inflammatory markers. It signals to a body that has been in survival mode that there is something worth surviving for.

I put rose petals on the windowsill when Dave came home. Not because I had read a study, though the studies exist. Because after six months of hospital corridors and antiseptic smell and the particular beige of medical facilities, I wanted something in our house that was unambiguously alive and beautiful. I wanted something that smelled like the world before all of this.

That instinct was not separate from the healing protocol. It was part of it.

The rose is the most written-about plant in human history. It appears in the oldest known perfume, excavated from a Bronze Age site in Cyprus dating to 1700 BCE. It is central to the medicine of Persia, where the physician Avicenna — Ibn Sina — included rose preparations extensively in his eleventh-century Canon of Medicine, one of the most influential medical texts ever written. It appears in the herbals of Hildegard of Bingen, in the Ayurvedic tradition as shatapatri, in Traditional Chinese Medicine as meigui hua. Every culture that has had access to roses has used them medicinally. Almost all of them used them, in part, for the heart.

The heart, in traditional medicine, was never purely a pump. It was the seat of emotion, of grief, of love and its losses. And rose, across every tradition that worked with it, was understood to speak to the heart in both senses simultaneously — the physical organ and the emotional one.

> *Modern research is beginning to confirm what traditional medicine always knew: the emotional heart and the physical heart are not separate systems, and a plant that addresses one is very likely addressing both.*

The active compounds in rose petals include a rich concentration of flavonoids — particularly quercetin, kaempferol, and anthocyanins — with documented antioxidant, anti-inflammatory, and cardioprotective properties. Rose petals are also a significant source of vitamin C, particularly in the form of rose hips, though the petals themselves contain meaningful amounts.

The essential oil, rose otto, contains geraniol, citronellol, and nerol — compounds with demonstrated antimicrobial, antispasmodic, and anxiolytic activity.

For Dave, whose cardiac event during his MICU stay remained a shadow on the recovery — a reminder that the heart had been under extraordinary stress — rose petals were a gentle, daily act of cardiovascular support. Not a replacement for his cardiology follow-up. Not a claim that a flower undoes what months of critical illness does to a heart. But a consistent, bioactive contribution to the conditions under which cardiac tissue heals and regenerates.

Beyond the cardiovascular, rose petals carry a specific affinity for grief. This is not poetry — or rather, it is both poetry and physiology simultaneously, which is what the best botanical medicine tends to be. The experience of prolonged crisis, of nearly losing someone, of six months of fear held in the body — that is a form of grief, even when the person survives. The body stores it. The nervous system carries it. And rose, with its gentle action on the limbic system — the brain's emotional processing center — has been used in every tradition that knew it to help the heart release what it has been holding.

Matthew Wood writes that rose is specific for "the person who has suffered a wound to the heart — literal or figurative — and needs gentle support in opening again." Avicenna prescribed rose preparations for sadness and palpitations in the same breath, understanding them as expressions of the same underlying condition.

There is a question I sat with often during those first months at home: who was healing whom? I was giving Dave the tinctures and making the teas and running the protocol. But the rose petals on the windowsill — those were also for me. For the part of me that had been holding six months of terror in my chest and needed, very quietly, to be allowed to let some of it go.

I think that is worth naming, for anyone reading this who is on the caregiver side of this story. The herbs are not only for the patient. The person who has been doing the holding needs tending too. Rose petals, in a cup of hot water, on a quiet morning, before the day begins — that is a small and legitimate act of self-restoration. Take it.

A Note on Sourcing Rose Petals

This matters more for rose than for almost any other herb in this reference, and I want to say it clearly: do not use rose petals from a florist, a grocery store bouquet, or any source that has not explicitly confirmed the flowers were grown without pesticides.

Commercially grown roses are among the most heavily pesticide-treated flowers in the agricultural industry. The rose you buy at a supermarket has almost certainly been treated with fungicides, insecticides, and preservatives that have no place in a medicinal preparation. They may be beautiful. They are not food. They are not medicine.

Source your rose petals from a certified organic grower, from a trusted small farm, or from your own garden — grown without chemical inputs, harvested in the morning when the dew has dried and the volatile oil content is highest, used fresh or dried immediately at low heat to preserve their compounds. The difference between a rose petal grown with care and one grown for the cut flower industry is not subtle. It is the difference between medicine and decoration.

The varieties most widely used medicinally are Rosa damascena (Damask Rose), Rosa centifolia (Cabbage Rose), and Rosa canina (Dog Rose, whose hips are used extensively). All three are available from reputable herb suppliers. When in doubt, Rosa damascena is the most thoroughly researched and most widely available in dried form from quality sources.

I put rose petals on the windowsill when Dave came home. A tincture from the farm, taken daily — for the gentle cardiovascular support, for the emotional dimension of a body that had been through something profound. Sometimes the body needs something as simple and ancient as a flower.

That is medicine too.

Body Systems: Cardiovascular | Nervous System | Immune | Emotional / Limbic

Ailments: Grief, Anxiety, Post-ICU Recovery, Cardiovascular Support, Immune Depletion, Caregiver Burnout, Emotional Trauma

Turmeric

Curcuma longa | The Golden Anti-Inflammatory

Turmeric is simultaneously one of the most studied medicinal plants in the world and one of the most misunderstood. It has been the subject of more than ten thousand published studies. Its primary active compound, curcumin, has been investigated for everything from cancer prevention to Alzheimer's disease to depression to inflammatory bowel disease — with results compelling enough to have attracted serious attention from pharmaceutical researchers who keep trying, and largely failing, to synthesize something that works as well.

And yet most people who "use" turmeric are doing so in a way that delivers almost none of its therapeutic benefit. A pinch of turmeric powder in a smoothie. A golden latte made with grocery store turmeric from a tin that has been sitting on the spice shelf for eighteen months. Curcumin consumed without fat, without black pepper, without the preparation methods that make it bioavailable — this is turmeric as color and flavor, not turmeric as medicine.

The difference matters enormously. And understanding it is the whole point of this profile.

In our household turmeric works two ways: as a tincture from the farm for concentrated therapeutic support, and as an ingredient in the kitchen — in the bone broth, in soups, in everything that simmers on a stove that has already decided food is medicine. Both approaches are intentional. Both are done with the bioavailability question in mind. And together they have been part of Dave's recovery from something that left systemic inflammation in nearly every system of his body.

Let me tell you what turmeric was addressing in a man who came home from six months in an MICU, because the list maps almost exactly to what curcumin has been most extensively studied for.

Systemic inflammation — because critical illness generates an inflammatory response so profound that it can persist for months or years after the acute event, contributing to fatigue, cognitive impairment, joint pain, and immune dysregulation long after the crisis has passed. Joint stiffness and pain — because prolonged immobility, steroid use, and the inflammatory burden of critical illness leave the joints carrying more than they should. Gut and digestive recovery — because the gut that has been through months of antibiotics, tube feeding, and pharmaceutical exposure needs anti-inflammatory support in the intestinal lining specifically. Liver support — because curcumin is hepatoprotective in ways that complement and extend the work of Milk Thistle and Burdock Root. And brain and cognitive function — because the post-ICU cognitive impairment that Dave experienced, the word that would not come and the train of thought that derailed, has a neuroinflammatory component that curcumin directly addresses.

> *Five distinct recovery needs. One root. That is not coincidence. That is a plant whose primary mechanism — the reduction of systemic inflammation through multiple simultaneous pathways — happens to be relevant to almost everything that prolonged critical illness leaves behind.*

The Science of Curcumin

Curcumin is a polyphenol — a class of plant compounds that interact with biological systems in ways that are complex, multi-targeted, and increasingly well understood. Its primary anti-inflammatory mechanism involves inhibition of NF-κB, a protein complex that acts as a master regulator of the inflammatory response — controlling the expression of genes that produce pro-inflammatory cytokines, enzymes, and adhesion molecules. When NF-κB is overactivated — as it is in chronic inflammatory conditions, in post-critical illness recovery, in the aftermath of prolonged infection — the body is essentially stuck in a low-grade inflammatory state that it cannot easily exit on its own.

Curcumin inhibits NF-κB activation through multiple mechanisms simultaneously, reducing the upstream signal rather than blocking individual downstream cytokines. This multi-target approach is why curcumin research shows relevance across such a wide range of inflammatory conditions — because it is addressing the master switch, not individual lights.

The anti-inflammatory evidence for Turmeric is among the strongest in botanical medicine — documented effects comparable to non-steroidal anti-inflammatory drugs in several conditions, without the gastrointestinal damage those drugs carry as standard side effects. The research is not preliminary. It is decades deep.

For the liver, curcumin's hepatoprotective effects have been documented in multiple studies, with mechanisms including reduction of oxidative stress in liver cells, inhibition of inflammatory signaling in hepatic tissue, and support of bile production that complements the silymarin activity of Milk Thistle. Used together, these two herbs address liver health from different and complementary angles — Milk Thistle protecting and regenerating liver cells,

Turmeric reducing the inflammatory environment in which those cells are working.

The Bioavailability Problem — And How to Solve It

Here is the conversation that most turmeric discussions skip, and it is the most practically important thing in this profile.

Curcumin is poorly absorbed from the digestive tract on its own. Studies on standard curcumin preparations show bioavailability as low as one percent — meaning that most of what you consume passes through the gut without entering the bloodstream in meaningful concentrations. The body cannot use what it cannot absorb. This is why people who add turmeric powder to food and expect therapeutic effects are often disappointed, and why researchers initially struggled to replicate in human trials the effects they observed in laboratory studies.

The solution has been known for centuries in Ayurvedic medicine, which combined turmeric with black pepper and fat as a matter of traditional practice long before anyone understood the biochemistry. Piperine — the active compound in black pepper — inhibits the intestinal enzyme and liver process that rapidly clears curcumin from the body, increasing bioavailability by up to 2,000 percent in some studies.

Fat increases absorption by making curcumin more soluble in the gut environment. These are not optional additions. They are the mechanism by which turmeric becomes medicine rather than spice.

> *When we cook with turmeric in this house — in the bone broth, in soups, in anything that simmers — black pepper goes in alongside it. Always. This is not a preference. It is the difference between turmeric as a beautiful golden color in your food and turmeric as something your body can actually use.*

A quality tincture from a trusted farm addresses the bioavailability problem through the extraction process itself — alcohol extraction in a properly made tincture delivers curcumin in a more bioavailable form than raw powder, and reputable farms formulate with bioavailability in mind. This is another reason why sourcing matters so fundamentally. A well-made turmeric tincture is not the same product as turmeric powder in a capsule, regardless of the curcumin percentage listed on the label.

Turmeric and the Post-ICU Brain

I want to spend a moment on the cognitive dimension of this herb, because it is the aspect of Dave's recovery that was hardest to watch and hardest to address, and because I think it is underrepresented in the conversation about what critical illness leaves behind.

Post-intensive care cognitive impairment is real, documented, and affects the majority of MICU survivors to some degree. It manifests as difficulty with memory, attention, processing speed, and executive function — the higher-order thinking that most of us rely on without noticing until it is not quite working as it should. For Dave it was subtle but present: the word that would not arrive when he reached for it, the task that required more concentration than it once had, the sense that his mind was moving through something slightly thicker than air.

The neuroinflammatory basis of this impairment — the inflammatory damage to brain tissue that occurs during critical illness and persists afterward — is the same mechanism that curcumin addresses through NF-κB inhibition and its antioxidant activity in neural tissue. I am not in a position to say that turmeric reversed Dave's cognitive symptoms. What I can say is that it was part of a protocol that addressed systemic inflammation comprehensively, and that over time the cognitive fog lifted in ways that were gradual, unannounced, and unmistakable.

One morning he used a word I had not heard him use in months — a specific, precise word that was just exactly right for what he was describing. He did not notice. I did. That is what recovery looks like when it is happening quietly, the way all the best healing does.

Turmeric worked two ways in our household — as a tincture from the farm for concentrated anti-inflammatory support, and in the kitchen every day in bone broth, soups, and everything that simmered. Always with freshly ground black pepper. Always. Without exception.

The golden root has been earning its place in the medicine chest of every culture that knew it for five thousand years. It has not changed. Only the preparation has. Get the preparation right, and you will understand why.

Body Systems: Immune | Liver & Gallbladder | Digestive | Neurological | Musculoskeletal

Ailments: Systemic Inflammation, Joint Pain, Post-ICU Recovery, Cognitive Impairment, Liver Support, Gut Inflammation, Arthritis, Neuroinflammation

Valerian

Valeriana officinalis | *For the Nervous System That Cannot Come Down*

I want to tell you something about the caregiver before I tell you about the herb.

There is a particular state that prolonged caregiving produces — something that is not quite anxiety in the ordinary sense and not quite exhaustion in the ordinary sense but is both of them at once, fused together into something the body wears like a second skin. You are tired in a way that sleep does not fully resolve. You are alert in a way that stillness does not fully quiet. Your nervous system has been running at maximum capacity for so long, responding to so many real emergencies with such sustained precision, that it has essentially forgotten how to idle.

When Dave came home from the hospital in September 2021, the crisis did not end. It changed shape.

The MICU had monitors. It had nurses. It had alarms that went off when something was wrong and staff who responded within seconds. Home had me. I slept right next to him — close enough to hear every breath, every shift in his breathing pattern, every cough that might mean something or might mean nothing and I had to know which. The pulse oximeter on the nightstand. The phone charged. One part of my nervous system permanently awake even when the rest of me was not, scanning the silence for anything that did not sound right.

The hypervigilance that had kept him alive during those six months did not have an off switch. It could not. I had trained myself to be always ready and my body did not know the emergency was over because in some ways it was not over. It was just quieter. He was breathing beside me instead of through a machine three miles away. But the listening never stopped.

> *The anxiety I was experiencing when Dave came home was outrageous. That is the only word that fits. Outrageous — meaning beyond what reason could contain, beyond what will alone could address, beyond what telling myself everything was fine could touch. My nervous system had its own knowledge and its own schedule and it was not consulting me.*

Valerian is the herb I reached for more than anyone else in this house. Not to sedate. Not to check out or go numb or stop paying attention — the man I loved was still on oxygen and I could not afford to stop paying attention. I reached for it to give a nervous system that had been running at emergency capacity for six months permission to come down without abandoning its post.

To find the difference between ready and braced. Between present and terrified.

That distinction — between an alert, present nervous system and a hypervigilant, exhausted one — is exactly what Valerian addresses. And understanding why requires understanding what the herb actually does.

What Valerian Does and How

Valerian root has been used as a sedative and anxiolytic herb for more than two thousand years. It appears in the writings of Hippocrates. Galen prescribed it for insomnia in the second century CE. It was used throughout medieval European medicine for nervousness, trembling, and the kind of anxiety that will not release its grip. By the First and Second World Wars it was being used by civilians in England and Germany to manage the stress of bombing raids — not as a pharmaceutical substitute but as the nervine herb it had always been, now pressed into service under conditions of collective trauma.

The primary active compounds in Valerian root are valerenic acid and its derivatives, along with isovaleric acid, a range of flavonoids including linarin and hesperidin, and alkaloids. The mechanism that has attracted the most research attention is valerenic acid's interaction with GABA receptors — the same receptor system targeted by benzodiazepine medications like Valium and Xanax.

GABA — gamma-aminobutyric acid — is the primary inhibitory neurotransmitter in the central nervous system. When GABA receptors are activated, the nervous system quiets. Anxiety decreases. Muscle tension releases. Sleep becomes accessible. Benzodiazepines work by binding to these receptors and forcing them open — an effective but blunt intervention that produces dependence, tolerance, and withdrawal effects that can be severe. Valerenic acid modulates GABA receptor activity through a different mechanism — not forcing the receptor open but enhancing the sensitivity of the receptor to the body's own GABA. The result is a gentler, more natural quieting of the nervous system, without the dependency profile, without the cognitive impairment, and without the rebound anxiety that benzodiazepine withdrawal produces.

The Caregiver's Nervous System

I want to stay with the caregiver for a moment because this book is read by caregivers, and the caregiver's nervous system is not a subject that appears in hospital discharge paperwork or post-ICU follow-up appointments. The patient gets the follow-up. The caregiver gets a handshake and a pamphlet.

What actually happens to a person who spends six months in acute crisis — driving to a hospital every day, making decisions under conditions of radical uncertainty, holding a family together while holding their own terror at bay — is a physiological event, not merely a psychological one. The sustained activation of the sympathetic nervous system, the months of elevated cortisol, the sleep disruption, the hypervigilance — these leave marks in the body that do not simply resolve when the crisis ends.

The research on caregiver health outcomes is sobering. Caregivers of critically ill patients show elevated rates of anxiety, depression, and PTSD that persist long after the patient's discharge. A study published in Critical Care Medicine found that nearly half of family caregivers of ICU survivors met criteria for clinically significant anxiety or depression at ninety days post-discharge, with many showing symptoms consistent with post-traumatic stress.

Nobody told me this. Nobody handed me a pamphlet about what six months of that kind of sustained crisis does to the person who holds everything together while the crisis is happening. I found my way to Valerian the same way I found my way to everything in this reference — by paying attention to what my body needed and going looking for what could help.

Sleeping next to someone you almost lost, listening to them breathe in the dark, is not the same as resting. It took time to learn the difference again. Valerian helped me find my way back to it.

Valerian and the Post-ICU Patient

While Valerian was primarily my herb during this period, its relevance to Dave's recovery is also real and worth naming. Post-intensive care syndrome — PICS — includes anxiety and sleep disruption as among its most consistent features. A nervous system that has been through five months of sedation, pain, delirium, and the particular terror of not being able to breathe is not a nervous system that simply returns to baseline when the acute event is over.

The GABA modulation that makes Valerian effective for anxiety and insomnia is relevant for post-ICU patients whose nervous systems are recalibrating after prolonged medical sedation — which works through many of the same GABA pathways. Gentle, non-habit-forming nervous system support during that recalibration period is exactly what Valerian offers. Used alongside Chamomile — which also works on GABA receptors through apigenin and which is covered in its own profile in this reference — the two herbs together provide broader and more sustained nervous system restoration than either alone.

The Chamomile and Oat Straw nervine blend in the Chamomile profile is designed for that daily restoration. Valerian is the targeted intervention for the nights when the nervous system needs more specific help coming down — when sleep will not arrive or anxiety will not release despite the gentler support.

A Note on the Smell

Valerian root smells terrible. I want to say this plainly because it surprises people the first time and I would rather prepare you than have you open the bottle and assume something has gone wrong.

The characteristic odor — earthy, pungent, reminiscent of old socks in the most charitable description — comes from isovaleric acid, one of the root's active compounds. It is a sign of quality and potency, not of spoilage. A Valerian tincture that smells strongly is a Valerian tincture that is working. A Valerian product with no smell at all should make you question its potency.

The smell dissipates in water. Taking it as a tincture in a small amount of water followed immediately by something with a stronger flavor — a sip of juice, a piece of fruit — makes it entirely manageable. It is one of the few herbs in this reference where the experience of taking it requires a small act of will. The sleep that follows is worth it.

*Valerian was primarily my herb during this period —
for the outrageous anxiety of a caregiver whose
nervous system did not know the emergency was over.
I used it in the evenings as a tincture from the farm.
Dave used it as well for the sleep disruption and
anxiety that are nearly universal in MICU survivors.*

*That is not a small thing. For a caregiver, that is
everything.*

Body Systems: Nervous System | Sleep | Adrenal | Emotional
*Ailments: Anxiety, Insomnia, Caregiver Stress, Post-Traumatic
Stress, Nervous System Overactivation, Post-ICU Recovery, Muscle
Tension, Wired Exhaustion*

Wild Lettuce

Lactuca virosa | *Nature's Pain Reliever*

There is a plant that the nineteenth century knew well and the twenty-first century has nearly forgotten. It was called lettuce opium. Not because it is an opiate — it is not — but because its effects on pain and anxiety were considered significant enough to earn the comparison, and to earn a place in the United States Pharmacopeia from 1820 to 1926, where it was listed as an official medicinal agent used by physicians across the country.

Then the pharmaceutical industry arrived with synthetic compounds that could be patented and sold at scale, and Wild Lettuce was quietly retired from the official record. Not because it stopped working. Because it could not be owned.

It still works. It has always worked. And for anyone managing pain — particularly nerve pain, the kind that burns and shoots and arrives without warning along pathways the body cannot seem to quiet — Wild Lettuce is one of the most important plants in this book.

I know this not only from the historical record, though the record is substantial. I know it because Dave used it. After six months in an MICU — after

ECMO and a tracheostomy and seventeen bronchoscopies and dialysis and a cardiac event and everything else that three pages of discharge paperwork documents — he developed shingles in the rehabilitation facility. Because of course he did. His immune system, depleted beyond what most bodies ever experience, finally let something through. The varicella-zoster virus, dormant in his nervous system like it is in anyone who has ever had chickenpox, saw its opening and took it.

The shingles rash appeared on his left side. The nerve pain that followed — post-herpetic neuralgia, the burning, persistent, treatment-resistant pain that travels the nerve pathways the virus inflamed — settled in his left foot, where it still visits occasionally, years later, as nerve pain tends to do.

> *Wild Lettuce tincture replaced pharmaceutical pain relief entirely for that nerve pain. Within an hour of taking it, the pain quiets. That is our experience. And in a body that could not afford one more pharmaceutical burden, that experience changed everything.*

I want to give you the science behind why, because Wild Lettuce deserves to be understood rather than simply trusted on faith — though faith, in this case, would be well placed.

What Wild Lettuce Actually Is

Lactuca virosa is a tall, branching plant in the daisy family, native to central and southern Europe and naturalized widely across North America. It is related to the common garden lettuce — Lactuca sativa — but considerably more potent medicinally, with a bitter white latex that oozes from cut stems and leaves. That latex, dried and collected, is lactucarium — the compound responsible for the plant's analgesic, sedative, and anxiolytic properties.

Lactucarium was used in European medicine for centuries before it appeared in American pharmacopeias. The ancient Egyptians associated wild lettuce with the god Min and used preparations of it ritually and medicinally. The Greek physician Dioscorides described its sedative properties in De Materia Medica in the first century CE. By the eighteenth and nineteenth centuries, European physicians were using lactucarium extensively as a cough suppressant, a sleep aid, and a pain reliever — particularly valued as an alternative to opium for patients in whom opium caused adverse effects or dependency.

A 2011 study confirmed significant sedative activity, with the compounds reducing spontaneous locomotor activity and potentiating sleep duration in ways consistent with central nervous system modulation.

Importantly, the mechanism appears to involve the same pain pathways targeted by conventional analgesics, without the opioid receptor binding that creates dependency.

For nerve pain specifically — the burning, electric, hypersensitive quality of post-herpetic neuralgia and other neuropathic conditions — Wild Lettuce's action on the central nervous system makes it particularly suited. Conventional medicine's primary pharmaceutical answer to neuropathic pain is gabapentin, which works by reducing nerve signal transmission broadly — a blunt instrument that brings cognitive fog, weight gain, dizziness, and a dependency profile that makes discontinuation difficult. Wild Lettuce appears to quiet the same signal through a different mechanism, without those costs.

This is a question worth sitting with: how many people are currently managing nerve pain with gabapentin or opioids — experiencing the fog, the weight, the dependence, the diminishment — who have never been told that a plant used by physicians for two centuries exists, and carries none of those burdens? I cannot answer that question. I can only tell you what I found, and what I observed.

Shingles, Nerve Pain, and the Exhausted Immune System

Shingles — herpes zoster — is caused by the reactivation of the varicella-zoster virus, which lies dormant in the dorsal root ganglia of the nervous system in anyone who has had chickenpox. In most people, the immune system keeps it suppressed indefinitely. Reactivation occurs when immune surveillance fails — under conditions of profound stress, illness, immunosuppression, or the natural decline of immune function with age.

After what Dave's immune system had been through, shingles was almost inevitable. Six months of sedation, mechanical ventilation, multiple courses of antibiotics and antivirals, immunosuppressive medications, dialysis, and the metabolic demands of critical illness had left his immune defenses at a fraction of their normal capacity. The virus recognized the opening. It travels along specific nerve pathways — in Dave's case, the nerves of the left thoracic region and down into the left foot — causing the characteristic blistering rash and the inflammation of the nerve tissue itself.

The rash resolves. The nerve damage, in many cases, does not — or at least not quickly. Post-herpetic neuralgia affects roughly 10 to 18 percent of shingles patients overall, and the rate is significantly higher in patients who were immunocompromised at the time of the outbreak. The pain can be constant or intermittent, triggered by light touch or temperature change, and can persist for months or years.

Dave's nerve pain is intermittent now — arriving in the left foot without much warning, along the pathway the virus carved. When it comes, the Wild Lettuce tincture is what he reaches for. Within an hour, in our experience, it quiets. He has not needed anything else for it. He has not had shingles again — which is, in its own quiet way, a testament to what rebuilding the immune system through food, herbs, clean environment, and reduced toxic load can accomplish over time.

For the Whole Family

Wild Lettuce is not only for nerve pain. Its analgesic and sedative properties make it useful across a wide range of pain presentations — headaches, muscular pain, the deep tension pain that accumulates in bodies under chronic stress, menstrual pain, joint pain, and the anxious, hypervigilant pain that has an emotional component woven through it, which most chronic pain does.

In our household it has been used by everyone at one point or another. A teenager with a bad headache. The muscle aches that come with a hard week. The kind of pain that used to mean reaching automatically for ibuprofen — which carries its own costs, including gastric lining damage, kidney stress, and cardiovascular effects with regular use that most people have never been told about.

I am not a physician and I am not suggesting Wild Lettuce is appropriate for every person or every pain situation. What I am saying is that in our experience, it has been effective, gentle, and free of the side effects we had come to accept as the unavoidable cost of pain relief. For a family that had already decided to question everything on the shelf, that mattered enormously.

Dave came home with pain in his feet and joints that was real and persistent. The reflexive answer would have been Tylenol or Advil — but after six months of pharmaceutical burden on his liver and kidneys, adding more was not something I was willing to do. Wild Lettuce tincture from the farm became our answer for pain management. Natural, effective, and without the organ cost.

That is not a prescription. That is a story. And sometimes a story is exactly what someone needs to go looking for their own answer.

Body Systems: Nervous System | Pain Response | Immune Support

Ailments: Nerve Pain, Post-Herpetic Neuralgia, Shingles Recovery, Chronic Pain, Headaches, Muscular Pain, Anxiety-Related Pain, Insomnia from Pain

Body Systems Index

This index organizes the herbs in this reference by the body systems they most directly support. It is designed to be used in two directions: if you know which system needs support, find it here and see which herbs address it. If you have already identified an herb you want to use, cross-reference its profile to understand which systems it serves.

A few things worth knowing before you use this index:

First, body systems do not operate independently. The liver depends on the lymphatic system to deliver what it needs to process. The nervous system and the gut communicate constantly through the vagus nerve. The immune system is housed, in large part, in the gut. Every system in this index influences and is influenced by the others, which is why multi-system herbs like Turmeric, Nettle, and Garlic appear across multiple categories.

Second, the herbs in this reference were chosen because they are the herbs that lived in this house, in this specific recovery, in this specific household. This is not a comprehensive botanical materia medica. It is a personal reference, grounded in one family's experience and supported by the research that explains what we observed. Other herbs exist. Other protocols exist. This is the one we know.

Third, the notes beneath each system are not instructions. They are the observations and practical connections that this particular protocol has produced. Use them as a starting point for your own thinking and your own conversation with a qualified practitioner.

Adrenal & Stress Response

Herbs that support the adrenal glands, cortisol regulation, and the body's physiological response to sustained stress.

Chamomile • Lemon Balm • Nettle • Valerian

Note: See also: Nervous System. Adrenal and nervous system support are deeply interconnected and many herbs serve both simultaneously.

Antimicrobial & Antiviral Defense

Herbs with documented activity against bacteria, viruses, fungi, and parasitic organisms — working with the immune system rather than replacing it.

Echinacea • Elderberry • Garlic • Isatis • Wild Lettuce

Note: See also: Immune System. The herbs in this category are most effective when combined with strong immune system support.

Antiparasitic Protocol

Herbs used in the antiparasitic cycling protocol described in Chapter Four. Each addresses parasitic organisms through a distinct mechanism — most effective used together.

Black Walnut Hull (Chapter Four) • Clove (Chapter Four) • Garlic • Wormwood (Chapter Four)

Note: Raw pumpkin seeds (Cucurbita pepo) are used alongside these herbs as the fifth agent in the protocol — see Chapter Four for the complete protocol and cycling schedule.

Cardiovascular & Circulatory

Herbs that support the heart muscle, blood pressure regulation, vascular integrity, endothelial health, and peripheral circulation.

Garlic • Ginger • Hawthorn • Rose Petals • Turmeric

Note: Hawthorn is the primary cardiac tonic in this reference. Rose Petals address the cardiovascular-emotional connection. Garlic and Turmeric work on vascular inflammation and blood pressure. Ginger supports peripheral circulation specifically.

Digestive System

Herbs that support digestion, gut motility, intestinal lining integrity, microbiome restoration, and the full range of digestive function from stomach to colon.
Burdock Root • Chamomile • Garlic • Ginger • Lemon Balm • Marshmallow Root • Milk Thistle • Turmeric

Note: For heartburn and reflux specifically: Ginger (motility) combined with Marshmallow Root (mucosal soothing). For post-antibiotic gut restoration: Burdock Root and Garlic. For the anxious gut: Lemon Balm and Chamomile.

Emotional & Psychological Support

Herbs that address the emotional and psychological dimensions of illness, recovery, grief, trauma, and the sustained stress of caregiving — recognized here as physiological realities, not secondary concerns.
Chamomile • Lemon Balm • Rose Petals • Valerian

Note: The emotional body and the physical body are not separate systems. Every herb in this reference that supports the nervous system also supports emotional wellbeing — this index simply names that dimension explicitly.

Gut-Brain Axis

Herbs that address the bidirectional communication between the enteric nervous system and the central nervous system — relevant wherever anxiety manifests as digestive symptoms or digestive dysfunction contributes to mood and cognition.

Chamomile • Ginger • Lemon Balm •
Marshmallow Root • Turmeric

Note: See also: Digestive System and Nervous System. The gut-brain axis is where those two systems meet — herbs that serve both are listed here for ease of navigation.

Immune System

Herbs that support, modulate, and restore immune function — including both the activation of immune response during illness and the restoration of immune capacity depleted by critical illness, prolonged stress, or pharmaceutical intervention.

Burdock Root • Chamomile • Echinacea •
Elderberry • Garlic • Ginger • Isatis • Milk
Thistle • Mullein • Nettle • Rose Petals •
Turmeric • Wild Lettuce

Note: For acute illness: Echinacea, Elderberry, and Isatis together as the Respiratory Illness Trinity. For post-ICU immune restoration: Nettle, Turmeric, and

Milk Thistle for the nutritional and inflammatory foundation.

Kidney & Urinary System

Herbs that support kidney filtration, urinary tract health, fluid balance, and the gentle ongoing support of kidneys that have carried significant burden.
Marshmallow Root • Nettle

Note: For post-dialysis kidney support: Nettle as the nutritional and tonic foundation, Marshmallow Root for urinary tract mucosal soothing. Both work slowly and require consistency over weeks and months.

Liver & Detoxification

Herbs that protect liver cells, support phase I and phase II liver detoxification, promote bile production and flow, and assist the liver in processing the pharmaceutical burden that critical illness treatment accumulates.
Burdock Root • Garlic • Milk Thistle • Turmeric

Note: Milk Thistle and Burdock Root are the liver support pair — most effective used together. Turmeric reduces hepatic inflammation alongside. Garlic supports detoxification through sulfur compounds. The three together provide comprehensive liver support.

Lymphatic System

Herbs that support lymphatic circulation, lymph node function, and the clearance of cellular waste and inflammatory debris — the drainage system that determines how efficiently the body clears what the immune system has identified.
Burdock Root • Echinacea • Mullein

Note: The lymphatic system has no pump of its own — it depends on movement, breath, and the gentle stimulation of herbs like these to maintain flow. Movement during the day, even gentle walking, works synergistically with lymphatic herbs.

Mucosal Lining & Tissue Repair

Herbs that coat, soothe, protect, and support the healing of mucous membranes throughout the body — from the esophagus and stomach through the intestinal tract, respiratory passages, and urinary tract.
Chamomile • Marshmallow Root • Mullein

Note: Marshmallow Root is the primary demulcent in this reference. Mullein addresses respiratory mucosal tissue specifically. Chamomile reduces mucosal inflammation through its anti-inflammatory flavonoids.

Musculoskeletal System

Herbs that address joint pain, muscle tension, inflammation in connective tissue, and the recovery of physical strength and mobility after prolonged immobility.

Ginger • Nettle • Turmeric • Wild Lettuce

Note: Turmeric and Ginger together address musculoskeletal inflammation from complementary angles. Wild Lettuce for pain with a nervous system component. Nettle for the nutritional support that tissue repair requires.

Nervous System

Herbs that calm, restore, and support the central and peripheral nervous system — addressing anxiety, hypervigilance, insomnia, and the nervous system dysregulation that both critical illness and prolonged caregiving produce.

Chamomile • Lemon Balm • Rose Petals •
Valerian • Wild Lettuce

Note: For daily gentle support: Chamomile and Lemon Balm. For acute intervention and sleep: Valerian. For pain with a nervous component: Wild Lettuce. For the emotional-nervous system connection: Rose Petals.

Neurological Support

Herbs with documented neuroprotective, anti-neuroinflammatory, or cognitive-supporting properties

— relevant for post-ICU cognitive impairment and the neurological sequelae of prolonged critical illness.
Lemon Balm • Turmeric • Wild Lettuce

Note: Post-intensive care cognitive impairment affects the majority of MICU survivors. Turmeric's NF-kB inhibition and blood-brain barrier penetration make it the primary neuroinflammatory herb in this reference. Lemon Balm supports cognitive calm and clarity.

Nutritional Support

Herbs that provide meaningful nutritional density — minerals, vitamins, amino acids, and trace elements that support the body's rebuilding process after the micronutrient depletion of critical illness.
Nettle • Rose Petals

Note: Nettle is the most nutritionally dense herb in this reference — complete protein, iron, calcium, magnesium, and silica in concentrations that rival pharmaceutical supplementation when prepared as a nourishing infusion.

Pain Response

Herbs that address pain through nervous system modulation, inflammation reduction, and the specific mechanisms of neuropathic and chronic pain — without the dependency profile of pharmaceutical analgesics.

Ginger • Turmeric • Wild Lettuce

Note: Wild Lettuce is the primary analgesic herb in this reference — specifically for nerve pain and post-herpetic neuralgia. Turmeric and Ginger address the inflammatory component of pain. For pain with sleep disruption, Wild Lettuce combined with Valerian.

Respiratory System

Herbs that support lung tissue, bronchial lining, respiratory immunity, and the slow restoration of respiratory capacity after ventilator dependence, chronic respiratory failure, or recurring respiratory illness.

Echinacea • Elderberry • Isatis • Marshmallow
  Root • Mullein • Nettle

Note: Mullein is the primary lung herb in this reference — begin here for any respiratory recovery. Add Elderberry and Echinacea for immune and antiviral support. Isatis for throat and upper respiratory infection specifically. Marshmallow Root for mucosal soothing throughout the respiratory tract.

Skin

Herbs that address skin conditions through the gut-lymph-skin axis — recognizing that most chronic skin conditions have a digestive or lymphatic root that topical treatment alone cannot resolve.

Burdock Root • Milk Thistle • Nettle

Note: The skin is an organ of elimination. When the gut and liver are overburdened, the skin becomes an auxiliary elimination route. Addressing skin conditions through Burdock Root and Milk Thistle for the liver and lymph, Nettle for the inflammatory component, produces more durable results than topical intervention alone.

Sleep

Herbs that support sleep onset, sleep quality, and the restoration of healthy sleep architecture — disrupted by critical illness, chronic pain, anxiety, and the hypervigilance of prolonged caregiving.

Chamomile • Lemon Balm • Valerian • Wild
  Lettuce

Note: For anxiety-driven insomnia: Valerian and Chamomile combined. For pain-driven insomnia: Wild Lettuce. For the racing mind that will not quiet: Lemon Balm in the evening followed by Valerian at bedtime. Consistency over weeks produces more durable results than single-dose use.

A note on the herbs that appear in Chapter Four but do not have standalone profiles in the herb reference: Black Walnut Hull, Wormwood, and Clove are covered in full in the context of the antiparasitic protocol. They are included in the Antiparasitic Protocol system above. For their full profiles, preparation details, and protocol context, see Chapter Four: Root Causes.

The body is not a collection of separate systems waiting to be treated separately. It is one integrated organism that heals as a whole when it is supported as a whole. Use this index to find entry points — and then follow the threads wherever they lead.

Ailment Index

This index is organized by symptom and situation — the way a person actually thinks when something is wrong. Find what you are experiencing, see which herbs address it, then turn to those profiles for the full context, preparation methods, and practical notes.

Herb names in bold indicate the primary herb for that ailment. Additional herbs listed alongside are supportive, complementary, or address the ailment through a different mechanism. Where a combination is specifically recommended, a note explains why.

This is not a diagnostic tool. It is a navigation aid through the herb profiles in this reference. For any serious, persistent, or acute medical condition, work with a qualified practitioner alongside whatever herbal support you choose to use.

ACUTE ILLNESS — When Something Is Coming On

Cold or Flu — First Sign

Echinacea • Elderberry • Isatis • Ginger

The Respiratory Illness Trinity at first sign: 30 drops each Elderberry, Echinacea, and Isatis every 3–4 hours for the first 24 hours. Add Ginger tea for warmth and immune support.

Fever

Isatis • Elderberry • Echinacea

Isatis is the primary herb for fever in the context of acute infection. Support with Elderberry and Echinacea for immune activation.

Throat Infection or Sore Throat

Isatis • Marshmallow Root

Isatis for the infection itself — antiviral and antibacterial. Marshmallow Root cold infusion for the inflamed mucosal tissue, sipped slowly throughout the day.

Upper Respiratory Infection

Isatis • Mullein • Echinacea • Elderberry

Isatis for targeted antiviral and antibacterial action in the respiratory tract. Mullein for the lung tissue. Echinacea and Elderberry for systemic immune support.

Bronchitis or Chest Congestion

Mullein • Isatis • Echinacea

Mullein is the primary herb — opens and soothes the bronchial passages. Add Isatis if infection is present, Echinacea for immune activation.

Influenza

Elderberry • Echinacea • Isatis • Ginger

Elderberry reduces influenza duration in clinical trials. Isatis has specific documented activity against influenza virus replication. Run the full Trinity protocol at maximum dose.

Immune Depletion — Recurring Illness

Echinacea • Elderberry • Nettle • Turmeric

Echinacea and Elderberry for immediate immune activation. Nettle and Turmeric for the nutritional and anti-inflammatory foundation that sustained immunity requires.

DIGESTIVE — Gut, Stomach, and Bowel

Nausea

Ginger

Fresh ginger root, one thin slice chewed slowly, is the fastest-acting preparation. Tincture in water for ongoing use. Repeat every 30 minutes as needed.

Heartburn or Acid Reflux

Ginger • Marshmallow Root

Always these two together: Ginger to improve gastric motility (addressing the cause), Marshmallow Root cold infusion to soothe the esophageal lining (addressing the tissue). Neither alone is as effective as both together.

Bloating and Gas

Ginger • Lemon Balm • Chamomile

Ginger for motility and movement. Lemon Balm and Chamomile for the smooth muscle tension that impedes it. Take 20–30 minutes before meals.

Digestive Sluggishness

Ginger • Lemon Balm • Burdock Root

Ginger is the prokinetic foundation. Lemon Balm for the nervous system component. Burdock Root for the lymphatic and liver support that sluggish digestion often reflects.

IBS — Irritable Bowel Symptoms

Chamomile • Lemon Balm • Marshmallow Root

Chamomile for digestive cramping and spasm. Lemon Balm for the gut-brain component — IBS is frequently a nervous system condition expressed through the gut. Marshmallow Root for mucosal lining support.

Nervous Stomach — Gut Anxiety

Lemon Balm • Chamomile

The anxious gut requires nervous system support, not just digestive support. Lemon Balm addresses the gut-brain axis directly. Chamomile relaxes smooth muscle and reduces the inflammatory response in the intestinal lining.

Digestive Cramping

Chamomile • Ginger

Chamomile is the primary antispasmodic. Ginger for the motility component. Together they address both the spasm and the sluggishness that often coexist.

Gut Lining Support — Leaky Gut, Inflammation

Marshmallow Root • Chamomile • Turmeric

Marshmallow Root coats and physically protects the intestinal lining. Chamomile reduces mucosal inflammation. Turmeric addresses the systemic inflammatory component.

Post-Antibiotic Gut Recovery

Burdock Root • Garlic • Ginger

Burdock Root's inulin content feeds the beneficial bacteria the antibiotics depleted. Garlic for the antimicrobial environment that prevents opportunistic organisms from filling the vacuum. Ginger to restore motility.

Post-Hospital Gut Recovery

Ginger • Lemon Balm • Marshmallow Root • Burdock Root

The gut after prolonged tube feeding needs motility restoration (Ginger), smooth muscle relaxation (Lemon Balm), mucosal healing (Marshmallow Root), and microbiome rebuilding (Burdock Root). All four, used consistently.

Liver Support — Ongoing

Milk Thistle • Burdock Root • Turmeric

The liver support trio. Milk Thistle protects and regenerates liver cells. Burdock Root supports lymphatic drainage and reduces the burden arriving at the liver. Turmeric reduces hepatic inflammation. Most effective used together daily.

Post-Pharmaceutical Liver Recovery

Milk Thistle • Burdock Root • Turmeric

Same trio, higher priority. After prolonged pharmaceutical exposure, begin with Milk Thistle and Burdock Root as a pair and add Turmeric within the first two weeks.

NERVOUS SYSTEM — Anxiety, Sleep, and Stress

Anxiety — General Daily

Lemon Balm • Chamomile

These two together for daily, sustained nervous system support that does not impair function. Take morning and afternoon. Most effective with consistent use over 2–4 weeks.

Anxiety — Acute or Heightened

Valerian • Lemon Balm • Chamomile

Add Valerian to the daily blend for acute periods. Valerian provides deeper GABA modulation without the dependency profile of pharmaceutical anxiolytics.

Caregiver Burnout and Stress

Valerian • Lemon Balm • Rose Petals • Nettle

Valerian for the nervous system that cannot come down. Lemon Balm for the daily background anxiety. Rose Petals for the emotional dimension. Nettle for the nutritional depletion that sustained stress produces. This is the caregiver's protocol.

Wired but Exhausted

Valerian • Chamomile

The specific state of being too tired to function and too activated to rest. Valerian and Chamomile combined in the early evening begins the process of bringing the nervous system down before sleep is even attempted.

Insomnia — Anxiety Driven

Valerian • Lemon Balm • Chamomile

Lemon Balm in the early evening to begin quieting the mind. Valerian 30–45 minutes before bed for deeper nervous system settling. Chamomile tea as the ritual that signals the body that the day is done.

Insomnia — Pain Driven

Wild Lettuce • Valerian

Wild Lettuce for the pain itself — analgesic action within one hour. Valerian alongside for the nervous system activation that pain produces and that prevents sleep even when the pain is managed.

Post-Traumatic Stress

Valerian • Lemon Balm • Rose Petals •
Chamomile

This is a full protocol, not a single herb situation. Valerian for the hypervigilant nervous system. Lemon Balm for the daily anxiety load. Chamomile for consistent gentle nervous system restoration. Rose Petals for the emotional and cardiac dimension of trauma.

Muscle Tension

Chamomile • Valerian • Wild Lettuce

Chamomile and Valerian for the nervous system tension that produces and sustains muscle tension. Wild Lettuce when tension has become pain.

CARDIOVASCULAR — Heart, Blood Pressure, and Circulation

High Blood Pressure

Hawthorn • Garlic • Turmeric • Rose Petals

Hawthorn is the primary antihypertensive herb in this reference. Garlic and Turmeric address the vascular inflammation that contributes to elevated pressure. Rose Petals for the endothelial dimension. All work gently over weeks — do not discontinue pharmaceutical management without practitioner guidance.

Post-Cardiac Event Recovery

Hawthorn • Rose Petals • Garlic • Turmeric

Hawthorn as the daily cardiac tonic. Rose Petals alongside for endothelial protection. Garlic and Turmeric for the vascular inflammatory environment. This is a long-term protocol — months, not weeks.

Poor Circulation — Cold Extremities

Ginger • Hawthorn

Ginger for immediate peripheral vasodilation and warming. Hawthorn for the underlying circulatory capacity that determines peripheral blood flow over time.

Heart Failure Support

Hawthorn

Hawthorn is the only herb in this reference with clinical trial data specifically for heart failure — the SPICE trial, 2,681 patients, 24 months. Use as a tonic alongside conventional medical management, not as a replacement for it.

Cardiovascular Endothelial Health

Hawthorn • Rose Petals • Turmeric • Garlic

The four herbs that collectively address endothelial lining integrity, vascular inflammation, and the oxidative stress that damages vessel walls over time.

RESPIRATORY — Lungs, Airways, and Breathing

Lung Recovery — Post-Ventilator or Chronic

Mullein

Begin here. Mullein tea from whole dried leaf, strained carefully, twice daily minimum. This is not an acute herb — it is the slow, consistent rebuilding of lung tissue and function that takes months and is worth every one of them.

Chronic Cough

Mullein • Marshmallow Root

Mullein for the bronchial and lung tissue. Marshmallow Root for the mucosal lining of the airways when the cough has an irritation component. Dry, irritating cough specifically benefits from Marshmallow Root cold infusion.

Seasonal Allergies

Nettle

Begin Nettle tincture 2-3 weeks before allergy season begins. Consistency and timing are more important than dose. Nettle inhibits histamine production upstream rather than blocking the receptor downstream — which is why it requires lead time and why it does not cause drowsiness.

Allergic Rhinitis

Nettle • Elderberry

Nettle as the primary antihistamine. Elderberry for the immune modulation that reduces the overreaction to environmental triggers.

Respiratory Vulnerability — Prone to Illness

Mullein • Elderberry • Echinacea

Mullein to strengthen the lung tissue itself. Elderberry and Echinacea for the immune surveillance that intercepts respiratory pathogens before they establish.

PAIN — Nerve, Joint, Muscle, and Chronic

Nerve Pain — Neuropathic

Wild Lettuce

The primary herb for nerve pain in this reference. Works through CNS modulation without opioid receptor binding. Tincture, 1–2 ml at onset, repeat after 2 hours if needed. Most effective for the sharp, burning quality of post-herpetic and neuropathic pain.

Post-Herpetic Neuralgia — Shingles Pain

Wild Lettuce

Wild Lettuce is the primary herb. The nerve pain of post-herpetic neuralgia — the lingering pain after shingles resolves — is the specific condition for which Wild Lettuce was used in this household with the most striking results.

Joint Pain and Arthritis

Turmeric • Ginger • Nettle

Turmeric and Ginger address the inflammatory mechanism. Nettle provides the mineral nutrition that joint tissue requires for repair. All three for sustained inflammatory joint conditions.

Muscle Pain

Wild Lettuce • Chamomile • Valerian

Wild Lettuce for the pain itself. Chamomile and Valerian for the muscle tension that accompanies and amplifies it.

Headaches

Wild Lettuce • Lemon Balm • Ginger

Wild Lettuce for the pain. Lemon Balm for the tension and anxiety component. Ginger for the circulatory component when headaches have a vascular quality.

Chronic Pain — Systemic Inflammation

Turmeric • Ginger • Wild Lettuce

Turmeric and Ginger for the inflammatory mechanism of chronic pain. Wild Lettuce for the pain itself when inflammation reduction alone is insufficient.

SKIN — Through the Gut-Lymph-Skin Axis

Chronic Skin Conditions — Eczema, Acne, Rashes

Burdock Root • Milk Thistle • Nettle

Skin conditions that recur despite topical treatment usually have a digestive or lymphatic root. Burdock Root and Milk Thistle for the liver and lymphatic system. Nettle for the inflammatory component. Allow 6–8 weeks of consistent use before assessing.

Skin as Elimination — Breakouts During Detox

Burdock Root • Milk Thistle

When the liver and lymphatic system are processing a significant burden, the skin often becomes an auxiliary elimination route. Burdock Root and Milk Thistle reduce that burden, which reduces the skin's need to assist.

KIDNEY AND URINARY — Filtration and Fluid

Urinary Tract Infection

Marshmallow Root • Nettle

Marshmallow Root cold infusion soothes the inflamed urinary tract lining and creates an environment less hospitable to bacterial adhesion. Nettle as the gentle diuretic that supports filtration and clearance. Drink both in large quantities alongside plain water.

Kidney Support — Ongoing

Nettle • Marshmallow Root

Nettle as the primary kidney tonic — gentle diuretic, mineral-rich, supportive of filtration without electrolyte stripping. Marshmallow Root for the mucosal lining of the urinary tract. Both for post-dialysis or any kidney history that warrants ongoing support.

Nutritional Depletion and Fatigue

Nettle • Rose Petals

Nettle nourishing infusion — steeped overnight — for the deepest mineral and nutritional restoration available from a plant source. Rose Petals alongside for the adrenal and emotional dimension of depletion that mineral supplementation alone does not address.

Anemia

Nettle

Nettle's iron content rivals animal sources when prepared as a long nourishing infusion. Begin with daily infusions steeped 4–8 hours. Allow 6–8 weeks of consistent use.

POST-ICU AND POST-HOSPITALIZATION RECOVERY

Post-Ventilator Lung Recovery

Mullein • Marshmallow Root • Elderberry

Mullein first, always. Marshmallow Root for the mucosal lining of airways that intubation has traumatized. Elderberry for the immune vulnerability of post-ICU lungs.

Post-ICU Cognitive Impairment — Brain Fog

Turmeric • Lemon Balm • Nettle

*Turmeric for the neuroinflammatory component —
the most direct anti-neuroinflammatory herb in this
reference. Lemon Balm for cognitive calm and clarity.
Nettle for the nutritional foundation that brain function
requires.*

Post-ICU Anxiety and Hypervigilance

Valerian • Lemon Balm • Chamomile — for the
  patient

*The same caregiver protocol applies to the patient
whose nervous system has been through critical
illness. PICS anxiety responds to the same gentle,
consistent nervous system support.*

Post-ICU Immune Restoration

Nettle • Echinacea • Elderberry • Turmeric

*Nettle for the nutritional foundation. Echinacea to
retrain immune activation. Elderberry to restore
antiviral defense. Turmeric for the systemic
inflammation that compromises immune function.
Introduce sequentially, not all at once.*

Post-Pharmaceutical Recovery

Milk Thistle • Burdock Root • Turmeric • Nettle

The liver trio plus Nettle for the nutritional rebuilding that pharmaceutical-intensive care depletes. This is the foundation protocol from which everything else builds.

Post-Dialysis Kidney Recovery

Nettle • Marshmallow Root

Nettle as the long-term kidney tonic. Marshmallow Root for urinary tract mucosal health. Both for the ongoing gentle support of kidneys that have carried the history of acute kidney injury.

Post-Intubation Throat and Esophageal Recovery

Marshmallow Root • Chamomile

Marshmallow Root cold infusion for the mucosal lining of the esophagus and throat that intubation and tracheostomy trauma. Chamomile for the inflammatory component. Sip slowly, frequently, throughout the day.

FOR THE CAREGIVER

This section is for the person who has been holding everything together. The one who drove sixty miles every day. Who slept next to someone on oxygen and called it rest. Who rebuilt the house and the kitchen and the protocol and still had to get up and do it again the next morning. Your body kept its own accounts during all of that. This section is for paying some of them back.

Caregiver Anxiety — The Background Hum

Lemon Balm • Chamomile

Daily, morning and afternoon, consistently. The anxiety that lives in the background of everything responds to consistency more than to dose.

Caregiver Exhaustion — Wired and Cannot Rest

Valerian • Chamomile

The specific exhaustion that coexists with hyperactivation. Valerian and Chamomile in the early evening, before the day ends, to begin the process of coming down.

Grief and Emotional Recovery

Rose Petals • Lemon Balm

Rose Petals for the heart — in every sense of that word. Lemon Balm for the nervous system and the gut where grief often lives. Both for the long, quiet work of coming back to yourself after something unsurvivable.

Nutritional Depletion from Sustained Stress

Nettle • Rose Petals

Sustained stress depletes magnesium, iron, B vitamins, and the trace minerals that the nervous system and immune system run on. Nettle nourishing infusion daily is the most direct nutritional restoration available from a plant source.

Anxiety in the Gut

Lemon Balm • Marshmallow Root • Ginger

The stress that lives in the stomach. Lemon Balm for the gut-brain axis. Marshmallow Root for the inflamed mucosal lining. Ginger for the motility that stress disrupts.

ANTIPARASITIC PROTOCOL — See Chapter Four

The full antiparasitic protocol — Black Walnut Hull, Wormwood, Clove, Garlic, and raw pumpkin seeds — is covered in complete detail in Chapter Four: Root Causes. The following is a navigation summary only.

Antiparasitic Protocol — Full Cycling Course

Black Walnut Hull • Wormwood • Clove • Garlic • Raw Pumpkin Seeds

See Chapter Four for the complete protocol, cycling schedule, and practical guidance. Support the liver throughout with Milk Thistle and Burdock Root.

Digestive Symptoms Without Clear Cause

Begin with Chapter Four

Bloating, irregularity, and gut discomfort that persist despite dietary and herbal digestive support may warrant the parasite question. Chapter Four addresses this directly.

Skin Issues Without Clear Cause

Burdock Root • Milk Thistle — then consider
  Chapter Four

Unexplained skin conditions that do not respond to the liver-lymph approach may have a parasitic component. See Chapter Four.

This index covers the ailments that lived in one household during one specific recovery. It is not exhaustive. It is honest. Use it as a starting point, follow the herb profiles for full context, and bring your questions to a practitioner willing to engage with them.

And if you receive the head tilt — find a different practitioner. Your questions are data. They deserve to be treated that way.

Building Your Home Apothecary

Start small. Start honest. Start wherever your body is telling you to start.

Before we talk about shelves and bottles and sourcing and storage, I want to say something that I wish someone had said to me at the beginning of all of this.

A simple rose petal and hawthorn tincture can be just as helpful as a cabinet full of seventeen herbs you do not fully understand yet.

Two bottles. One for the heart that has been through something. One for the emotional weight of what it means to love someone through a crisis. Both chosen with intention. Both understood. Both used consistently. That is not a starter kit waiting to become something real. That is already something real.

The home apothecary I have now did not arrive all at once. It was built one bottle at a time, in response to one need at a time, over months of paying attention to what was working and what was still missing. The shelf I have today is the record of a learning process, not the implementation of a plan. And every herb on it earned its place by doing something specific for someone specific in this household.

Alongside the tinctures, I keep my favorite herbs in dried form. Mullein for a tea when someone's chest is heavy. Chamomile for an evening when the day has been too much. Rose petals in a jar because they are beautiful and beauty is medicine and sometimes a cup of rose petal tea is exactly the right thing. Because who doesn't just like a hot tea?

That is the honest version of my apothecary. A dedicated shelf. Tinctures from people I trust. Dried herbs for the tea that a hard day sometimes calls for more than anything else. It is not complicated. It does not need to be.

The Only Rule That Matters

Start wherever your body is telling you to start.

Not where a list tells you to start. Not where the most comprehensive protocol begins. Not at the beginning of this reference or the end of it. Wherever the need is loudest, wherever the symptom is most persistent, wherever the question has been living rent-free in your thinking for longer than you want to admit — start there.

Because the herb you choose because you understand why you need it is worth ten herbs chosen because someone told you they belonged in a well-stocked apothecary. Understanding is the difference between a supplement you remember to take and one that sits unopened on the shelf next to all the other unopened supplements that were supposed to help.

The body is always telling you something. The home apothecary is the practice of learning to hear it and having something useful to reach for when you do.

Four Principles Worth Keeping

These are not rules. They are what I would tell someone standing in front of their first empty shelf, trying to figure out where to begin, and feeling the faint anxiety of not knowing enough yet.

One: Quality over quantity. Always.

- Two good tinctures from a farm you trust will do more than ten bottles from a supplement company that sources from the lowest bidder.

A tincture is only as good as the plant it was made from, the soil that plant grew in, the moment it was harvested, and the care taken in extraction. None of those things appear on a label. They appear in what you feel when you take it.

Two: Buy from people who grow what they sell.

- The herb reference in this book makes repeated reference to the farm because the farm is not incidental to the protocol. It is the protocol.

A person who grows Echinacea, harvests it at peak alkamide content, and makes the tincture themselves knows something about that plant that a manufacturer producing ten thousand units a week does not. Find those people. Build that relationship. It will change what you think herbal medicine is capable of.

Three: Store properly or don't bother.

- Cool, dark, away from heat sources and direct light. A dedicated shelf or cabinet that stays closed.

Light and heat degrade the active compounds in tinctures faster than almost anything else. A tincture stored in a sunny windowsill or on a shelf above the stove is a tincture losing its potency every day. The dark glass bottle is not an aesthetic choice. It is functional. Keep it somewhere dark and it will last years. Keep it somewhere bright and warm and it will be half the product within months.

Four: Start small and build as you learn.

- An apothecary that grows with your understanding is an apothecary you will actually use.

Resistance to herbal medicine often comes not from the herbs themselves but from the overwhelm of trying to implement too much at once without the understanding that makes it sustainable. Start with one or two herbs. Learn them. Use them until you know how they work in your body and your household. Then add the next one. The knowledge compounds the same way the herbs do — slowly, quietly, with results that show up before you realize the accumulation has happened.

What a Starting Shelf Might Look Like

The following are not prescriptions. They are suggestions organized by situation — the most common entry points into herbal medicine that the profiles in this book address. Choose the one that matches where you are. The rest will follow in its own time.

If you are supporting someone in post-ICU or post-hospitalization recovery:

- Mullein tincture — for the lungs, always first

- Milk Thistle tincture — for the liver carrying the pharmaceutical burden
- Burdock Root tincture — for the lymphatic system and microbiome rebuilding
- Chamomile dried herb — for the evening, for the nervous system, for the sleep that comes in fragments
- Nettle dried herb — steeped overnight for the deepest nutritional restoration

If your primary concern is immune support for the whole family:

- Elderberry tincture — the first thing out at any sign of illness
- Echinacea tincture — alongside Elderberry, always together
- Isatis tincture — when illness moves into the throat or respiratory tract
- Garlic — in the kitchen, crushed and rested, in everything savory

If you are a caregiver managing sustained anxiety and depletion:

- Lemon Balm tincture — daily, morning and afternoon, for the background hum
- Valerian tincture — for the evenings when the nervous system cannot come down

- Rose Petals dried herb — because beauty is medicine and you have earned a cup of something lovely
- Nettle dried herb — for the nutritional depletion that sustained stress produces

If you are addressing cardiovascular recovery:

- Hawthorn tincture — the daily cardiac tonic, taken consistently for months
- Rose Petals tincture — alongside Hawthorn, for the endothelial and emotional dimensions
- Garlic — in the tincture and in the kitchen, both
- Turmeric — in the tincture and in the bone broth with black pepper, always

If you are beginning with just two things — start here:

- Rose Petals and Hawthorn.

For the heart. For the person you love. For the weight of what both of you have been through. Two bottles. Understood. Intentional. Enough to begin.

The Kitchen Is Part of the Apothecary

This deserves its own moment because it is easy to think of the apothecary as the shelf and the kitchen as something separate. In this house they are not separate. They are the same intention expressed through different forms.

Celtic sea salt in everything cooked — for the minerals. Black pepper in everything savory — for the piperine that makes turmeric and every other fat-soluble compound bioavailable. Garlic crushed and rested before it meets heat. Turmeric in the bone broth. Ginger in the soup. These are not cooking preferences. They are the daily protocol that runs underneath the tinctures, reinforcing them, extending them, making every meal a small continued act of the same intention the shelf represents.

The exception is baking. The cake does not need black pepper. Some things are just cake.

But everything else — everything savory, everything simmered, everything that comes out of a pot or a pan in this kitchen — carries the same philosophy as every bottle on the shelf. Food as medicine. Intention as practice. The kitchen and the apothecary as one continuous space organized around the same question: what does this body need, and what do I have that can help?

Go to Your Local Herb Farm

I want to tell you something directly, the way I would tell a friend: go to your local herb farm. Just go. Walk in and look at what they have.

See what herbal tinctures they carry. Trust me — there are a lot. More than you expect. More than you knew existed. And they are right there, grown by people who know them, made by hands that understand what they are doing, available to you without a prescription or an appointment or anyone's permission.

Pick up the ones whose names you do not recognize. Look them up when you get home. Read what they help, what they heal, what traditions they come from and what the research says about them. Let yourself be surprised by how much exists that nobody ever told you about. Let the curiosity pull you wherever it pulls you.

You will not regret it. I promise you that. The person who walks into an herb farm for the first time and starts asking questions is not the same person who walks out. Something shifts — quietly, without announcement — in the direction of agency. Of the understanding that there are more options available to you than the ones that have been presented to you. That healing has a longer history and a wider vocabulary than any single system of medicine contains.

The farm is where this book began for me — not the writing of it, but the living of it. The first tincture I brought home. The first conversation with someone who grew what they were selling and could tell me exactly when it was harvested and why that mattered.

That conversation changed the direction of everything that followed.

Go find yours. It is waiting for you. And so is everything you are going to learn once you walk through the door.

On Making Your Own

If you want to learn to make tinctures, teas, infusions, and decoctions yourself — that knowledge is worth having. Not because it is necessary, but because understanding how a preparation is made changes the way you understand what it does. There is something that happens when you pack a mason jar with fresh plant material, cover it with alcohol, label it with the date, and wait — something that is partly practical and partly a relationship with the plant that the finished bottle from a farm does not quite replicate.

The resources for learning this well are available. Rosemary Gladstar's Medicinal Herbs: A Beginner's Guide is the most accessible entry point in print — clear, practical, written by someone who has been teaching this for decades and who understands that the goal is confidence, not complexity. Susun Weed's Healing Wise goes deeper into the philosophy of plant relationship and the nourishing herbal infusion tradition that Nettle and other tonic herbs belong to.

But do not let the desire to eventually make your own become a reason to wait. The tincture from the farm is real medicine today. The knowledge of how to make it is a project for a quieter season, when the crisis has passed and the learning can happen without urgency.

Buy what makes sense now. Learn what you can when you can. The shelf does not judge the source of what is on it. It only cares whether it is good and whether you understand why it is there.

A Final Word on This Shelf

The apothecary I have built did not come from a plan. It came from a crisis, and from the months of reading and learning and paying attention that a crisis made necessary. It came from a man on oxygen in the next room and two daughters watching their mother figure out how to help him. It came from sixty miles of driving and four hours at a hospital bedside and the long, quiet evenings after, when the house was finally still and I could think.

I did not set out to build a medicine cabinet. I set out to help one person get better. The cabinet is what happened along the way, as each new question led to each new herb, as each herb earned its place by doing something real for someone real in this house.

That is the only apothecary worth building. Not the one from the list. The one from the need. The one that grew out of paying attention to a specific body in a specific recovery and asking, each time: what does this body need right now, and do I have something that can help?

> *Start with two bottles if that is where you are. Start with rose petals and hawthorn if your heart — or someone else's — is what needs tending. Start with the immune protocol if illness is what you are up against. Start with the caregiver herbs if the person who most needs support right now is you.*

Start somewhere. The body is waiting. And it already knows, before you do, exactly where to begin.

The shelf in my house holds what this family has needed. Your shelf will hold what yours needs. Those will not be identical lists, and they should not be. The home apothecary is not a standard formula. It is a personal practice, built from attention and love and the willingness to ask better questions than the ones you were given.

That willingness — more than any herb on any shelf — is where all of this begins.

References

Chapters One Through Four

Steinemann A.C., Fragranced consumer products and undisclosed ingredients, Environmental Impact Assessment Review, 29(1), 2009

Flegr J., Effects of Toxoplasma on human behavior, Schizophrenia Bulletin, 33(3), 2007

Centers for Disease Control and Prevention, Parasites — About Parasitic Diseases, Division of Parasitic Diseases and Malaria, 2023

Environmental Working Group, Skin Deep Cosmetics Database, ewg.org/skindeep (ongoing database, first published 2004)

Robin Wall Kimmerer, Braiding Sweetgrass: Indigenous Wisdom, Scientific Knowledge, and the Teachings of Plants (Milkweed Editions, 2013)

Rosemary Gladstar, Rosemary Gladstar's Medicinal Herbs: A Beginner's Guide (Storey Publishing, 2012)

Milk Thistle

Dr. Aviva Romm, Botanical Medicine for Women's Health (Churchill Livingstone, 2010)

Mark Blumenthal, Herbal Medicine: Expanded Commission E Monographs (American Botanical Council, 2000)

Eunice D. Ingham, Stories the Feet Can Tell Thru Reflexology (Ingham Publishing, 1938; updated edition available through the International Institute of Reflexology)

Needham D.M. et al., Improving long-term outcomes after discharge from intensive care unit, Critical Care Medicine, 40(2), 2012 — foundational paper establishing Post-Intensive Care Syndrome (PICS)

Pandharipande P.P. et al., Long-term cognitive impairment after critical illness, New England Journal of Medicine, 369(14), 2013

Alcock J. et al., Is eating behavior manipulated by the gastrointestinal microbiota? Evolutionary pressures and potential mechanisms, BioEssays, 36(10), 2014

Vighi G. et al., Allergy and the gastrointestinal system, Clinical and Experimental Immunology, 153(S1), 2008

Steenland K. et al., Epidemiologic evidence on the health effects of perfluorooctanoic acid (PFOA), Environmental Health Perspectives, 118(8), 2010

Vallejo F. et al., Phenolic compound contents in edible parts of broccoli inflorescences after domestic cooking, Journal of the Science of Food and Agriculture, 83(14), 2003

Cos P. et al., Juglone: Activity against Trypanosoma and Leishmania species, Phytomedicine, 9(1), 2002

Efferth T. et al., The antiviral activities of artemisinin and artesunate, Clinical Infectious Diseases, 47(6), 2008

Tragoolpua Y., Jatisatienr A., Anti-herpes simplex virus activities of Eugenia caryophyllus oil and eugenol, Phytotherapy Research, 21(12), 2007

Burdock Root

Predes F.S. et al., Antioxidative and in vitro antiproliferative activity of Arctium lappa root extracts, BMC Complementary and Alternative Medicine, 11(25), 2011

David Hoffmann, Medical Herbalism: The Science and Practice of Herbal Medicine (Healing Arts Press, 2003)

Kiani A.K. et al., Prevalence of intestinal parasitic infections in Europe: a systematic review, Parasitology Research, 2022

Chamomile

Matthew Wood, The Earthwise Herbal: A Complete Guide to Old World Medicinal Plants (North Atlantic Books, 2008)

Amsterdam J.D. et al., A randomized, double-blind, placebo-controlled trial of oral Matricaria recutita (chamomile) extract therapy for generalized anxiety disorder, Journal of Clinical Psychopharmacology, 29(4), 2009

Mao J.J. et al., Long-term chamomile therapy of generalized anxiety disorder: A randomized clinical trial, Phytomedicine, 23(14), 2016

Bienvenu O.J. et al., Posttraumatic stress disorder symptoms after acute lung injury: a 2-year prospective longitudinal study, Psychological Medicine, 43(12), 2013

Echinacea

A comprehensive meta-analysis published in Lancet Infectious Diseases in 2015, analyzing 24 randomized trials involving more than 4,000 participants, found that Echinacea preparations reduced the incidence of the common cold by 35 percent and reduced the duration of colds by 1.4 days on average. The authors noted that effects were most pronounced with higher-quality preparations and with use initiated at the earliest signs of infection.

Karsch-Völk M. et al., Echinacea for preventing and treating the common cold, Cochrane Database of Systematic Reviews, 2, 2015

Isatis

Deng L. et al., Antiviral effects of Radix Isatidis on influenza viruses, Chinese Medical Journal, 123(18), 2010

Hamburger M. et al., Isatis tinctoria — from the rediscovery of an ancient medicinal plant towards a novel anti-inflammatory phytopharmaceutical, Phytochemistry Reviews, 1(3), 2002

Elderberry

Tiralongo E. et al., Elderberry supplementation reduces cold duration and symptoms in air-travellers: A randomized, double-blind placebo-controlled clinical trial, Nutrients, 8(4), 2016

A 2004 study in the Journal of International Medical Research
found that elderberry extract reduced the duration of
influenza by an average of four days compared to placebo,
with patients reporting significantly faster relief of symptoms
including fever, headache, muscle aches, and nasal
congestion.

Zakay-Rones Z. et al., Randomized study of the efficacy and safety
of oral elderberry extract in the treatment of influenza A and
B virus infections, Journal of International Medical Research,
32(2), 2004

Barak V. et al., The effect of Sambucol, a black elderberry-based
natural product, on the production of human cytokines,
European Cytokine Network, 12(2), 2001

A 2020 review in the Journal of Functional Foods examined the
available evidence specifically on this question and concluded
that there was no clinical evidence supporting the concern
that elderberry use increases the risk of cytokine storm, and
that the theoretical basis for the concern was not well
supported by the mechanistic research on how elderberry
actually interacts with immune function.

Hawkins J. et al., Black elderberry (Sambucus nigra)
supplementation effectively treats upper respiratory
symptoms: A meta-analysis of randomized, controlled clinical
trials, Complementary Therapies in Medicine, 42, 2019

Garlic

Ankri S., Mirelman D., Antimicrobial properties of allicin from
garlic, Microbes and Infection, 1(2), 1999

Caili F. et al., A review on pharmacological activities and
utilization technologies of pumpkin, Plant Foods for Human
Nutrition, 61(2), 2006

Rosemary Gladstar, Rosemary Gladstar's Medicinal Herbs: A
Beginner's Guide (Storey Publishing, 2012)

Susun S. Weed, Healing Wise (Ash Tree Publishing, 1989)

A meta-analysis published in the Journal of Nutrition analyzing
eleven randomized controlled trials found that garlic
supplementation produced a significant reduction in systolic
and diastolic blood pressure compared to placebo, with effects
most pronounced in participants with elevated baseline blood
pressure — the population for whom it matters most.

Ried K. et al., Effect of garlic on blood pressure: A systematic
review and meta-analysis, BMC Cardiovascular Disorders,
8(13), 2008

Harris J.C. et al., Antimicrobial properties of Allium sativum,
Applied Microbiology and Biotechnology, 57(3), 2001

Hawthorn

A landmark clinical trial — the SPICE trial, published in the
European Journal of Heart Failure in 2008 — followed 2,681
patients with heart failure over 24 months and found that
Hawthorn extract produced significant improvement in
exercise tolerance and significant reduction in symptoms
including shortness of breath and fatigue, with an excellent
safety profile and no adverse interactions with standard
cardiac medications.

Holubarsch C.J. et al., The efficacy and safety of Crataegus extract
WS 1442 in patients with heart failure, European Journal of
Heart Failure, 10(12), 2008

A meta-analysis published in the American Journal of Medicine
analyzing fourteen randomized controlled trials concluded
that Hawthorn extract produced significant improvements in
exercise tolerance, significant reductions in shortness of
breath and fatigue, and a reduction in resting blood pressure
across the studies reviewed.

Pittler M.H. et al., Hawthorn extract for treating chronic heart
failure, American Journal of Medicine, 114(8), 2003

For blood pressure specifically, Hawthorn's antihypertensive
effects work through vasodilation and reduction of peripheral
resistance rather than through the aggressive mechanisms of

pharmaceutical antihypertensives — which means they work
gently and without the side effects of fatigue, electrolyte
disruption, and sexual dysfunction that many pharmaceutical
blood pressure medications produce. A pilot study published
in the British Journal of General Practice found that Hawthorn
extract produced significant reductions in diastolic blood
pressure in patients with type 2 diabetes, with no adverse
effects reported.

Walker A.F. et al., Promising hypotensive effect of hawthorn
extract, British Journal of General Practice, 52(484), 2002

Ginger

Viljoen E. et al., A systematic review and meta-analysis of the
effect and safety of ginger in the treatment of pregnancy-
associated nausea and vomiting, Nutrition Journal, 13(20),
2014

For circulation, ginger's warming properties — the ones that
make it indispensable in cold climates and cold seasons — are
driven by its ability to increase peripheral circulation, dilate
blood vessels, and improve blood flow to the extremities. Cold
hands and feet that do not respond to simply warming up are
often a circulation issue, and ginger addresses that directly. A
clinical study published in the Journal of Nutrition found that
ginger supplementation significantly reduced markers of
cardiovascular inflammation and improved circulatory
parameters in participants with metabolic syndrome.

Arablou T. et al., The effect of ginger consumption on glycemic
status, lipid profile and some inflammatory markers in
patients with type 2 diabetes, International Journal of Food
Sciences and Nutrition, 65(4), 2014

Ginger's prokinetic properties — its ability to stimulate and
normalize gut motility — make it particularly relevant for
exactly this situation. A study published in the European
Journal of Gastroenterology and Hepatology found that ginger
significantly accelerated gastric emptying and improved
symptoms of functional dyspepsia — the category of digestive

239

dysfunction that includes the post-hospitalization gut sluggishness Dave experienced.

Hu M.L. et al., Effect of ginger on gastric motility and symptoms of functional dyspepsia, World Journal of Gastroenterology, 17(1), 2011

Marshmallow Root

Fink C. et al., Efficacy and tolerability of a fluid extract combination of thyme herb and ivy leaves and matched placebo in adults suffering from acute bronchitis, Arzneimittelforschung, 2006

Deters A. et al., Aqueous extracts and polysaccharides from Marshmallow roots inhibit the adherence of Helicobacter pylori to human gastric mucosa, Journal of Ethnopharmacology, 125(2), 2010

Lemon Balm

Cases J. et al., Pilot trial of Melissa officinalis L. leaf extract in the treatment of volunteers suffering from mild-to-moderate anxiety disorders and sleep disturbances, Mediterranean Journal of Nutrition and Metabolism, 4(3), 2011

Madisch A. et al., Treatment of functional dyspepsia with a herbal preparation, Digestion, 69(1), 2004

Mullein

Research published in the Journal of Ethnopharmacology has confirmed significant antimicrobial activity in Mullein leaf extracts against several respiratory pathogens, including Klebsiella pneumoniae and Staphylococcus aureus — the kinds of bacteria that colonize already-compromised lung tissue. A study in the same journal documented activity against Mycobacterium tuberculosis, the pathogen responsible for tuberculosis, long treated with Mullein in folk traditions before the mechanism was ever understood.

Turker A.U., Camper N.D., Biological activity of common mullein, a medicinal plant, Journal of Ethnopharmacology, 82(2-3), 2002

Susun S. Weed, Healing Wise (Ash Tree Publishing, 1989)

Nettle

A randomized double-blind study published in Planta Medica found that freeze-dried Nettle leaf was rated moderately to highly effective by 58 percent of participants in reducing allergy symptoms, compared to 37 percent in the placebo group, with participants rating it comparable to over-the-counter allergy medications but without the drowsiness and cognitive side effects.

Mittman P., Randomized, double-blind study of freeze-dried Urtica dioica in the treatment of allergic rhinitis, Planta Medica, 56(1), 1990

A landmark study published in JAMA Internal Medicine in 2015 found that cumulative use of anticholinergic medications, including first-generation antihistamines like diphenhydramine, was associated with a significantly increased risk of dementia, with higher cumulative doses associated with higher risk. The relationship was dose-dependent and persisted after controlling for other risk factors.

Gray S.L. et al., Cumulative use of strong anticholinergics and incident dementia, JAMA Internal Medicine, 175(3), 2015

Susun S. Weed, Healing Wise (Ash Tree Publishing, 1989)

Nettle is a gentle diuretic — it increases urine output and supports the kidney's filtration function without the electrolyte stripping that pharmaceutical diuretics produce. It reduces inflammation in the urinary tract, supports the clearance of uric acid and other metabolic waste products, and has been used in both European and Ayurvedic medicine for kidney and urinary conditions for centuries. A review published in Phytotherapy Research documented Nettle's anti-inflammatory and diuretic mechanisms and noted its traditional use for kidney support across multiple medical traditions.

Chrubasik J.E. et al., A comprehensive review on the stinging nettle effect and efficacy profiles, Phytotherapy Research, 21(7), 2007

Rose Petals

Matthew Wood, The Earthwise Herbal: A Complete Guide to Old World Medicinal Plants (North Atlantic Books, 2008)

A 2011 study published in Phytomedicine found that Rosa damascena extract produced significant reductions in anxiety and pain perception. Research published in the Iranian Journal of Basic Medical Sciences documented anti-inflammatory effects comparable in some measures to non-steroidal anti-inflammatory drugs, without the gastrointestinal side effects. A growing body of research on rose flavonoids confirms cardioprotective activity — reducing oxidative stress in cardiac tissue, supporting healthy blood pressure, and protecting the endothelial lining of blood vessels.

Boskabady M.H. et al., Pharmacological effects of Rosa damascena, Iranian Journal of Basic Medical Sciences, 14(4), 2011

Turmeric

For the brain specifically, a randomized, double-blind, placebo-controlled trial published in the American Journal of Geriatric Psychiatry in 2018 found that bioavailable curcumin supplementation over 18 months produced significant improvements in memory and attention in adults without dementia, along with reductions in amyloid and tau levels in brain regions associated with memory and emotional regulation. The authors noted that the anti-inflammatory and antioxidant properties of curcumin likely underlie these cognitive effects.

Small G.W. et al., Memory and brain amyloid and tau effects of a bioavailable form of curcumin in non-demented adults: A double-blind, placebo-controlled 18-month trial, American Journal of Geriatric Psychiatry, 26(3), 2018

Rahmani A.H. et al., Curcumin: A potential candidate in prevention of cancer via modulation of molecular pathways, BioMed Research International, 2014

Shoba G. et al., Influence of piperine on the pharmacokinetics of curcumin in animals and human volunteers, Planta Medica, 64(4), 1998

Valerian

A meta-analysis published in the American Journal of Medicine reviewing sixteen randomized controlled trials found that Valerian improved sleep quality without producing side effects, with the most consistent benefits seen in subjective measures of sleep onset, sleep quality, and morning alertness — the last being particularly relevant for a caregiver who needed to be functional and present the next day, not foggy from a sedative.

Bent S. et al., Valerian for sleep: A systematic review and meta-analysis, American Journal of Medicine, 119(12), 2006

For anxiety specifically, a randomized controlled trial published in Phytotherapy Research found that Valerian extract produced significant reductions in anxiety symptoms in participants with generalized anxiety disorder, with effects comparable to diazepam — a benzodiazepine — but without the sedation, cognitive impairment, or withdrawal effects associated with that medication.

Andreatini R. et al., Effect of valepotriates on the cognitive and psychomotor performance of healthy volunteers, Phytotherapy Research, 16(7), 2002

Davidson J.E. et al., Post-intensive care syndrome: What it is and how to help prevent it, American Journal of Nursing, 113(11), 2013

Wild Lettuce

The primary active compounds in lactucarium are lactucin and
lactucopicrin — sesquiterpene lactones with documented
analgesic and sedative activity. A landmark study published in
the Journal of Ethnopharmacology in 2006 found that lactucin
and lactucopicrin produced analgesic effects comparable to
ibuprofen in animal models, with lactucopicrin showing
activity approaching that of morphine at higher doses —
without the respiratory depression, dependency profile, or
gastrointestinal damage associated with either
pharmaceutical.

Wesołowska A. et al., Analgesic and sedative activities of lactucin
and some lactucin-related compounds from Lactuca virosa L.,
Journal of Ethnopharmacology, 107(2), 2006

Yakoot M., Salem A., Helmy S., A pilot study of the efficacy and
safety of lettuce seed oil in patients with sleep disorders,
International Journal of General Medicine, 4, 2011

Volpi A. et al., Worst cases of herpes zoster, American Journal of
Clinical Dermatology, 9(4), 2008

www.ingramcontent.com/pod-product-compliance
Lightning Source LLC
Chambersburg PA
CBHW072009170726
47999CB00014B/1369